SETTING THINGS
Straight

Achieving Spectacular Health Without
Medical Guesswork, Drastic Dieting and Deadly Drugs

JOHN MADEIRA, D.C.

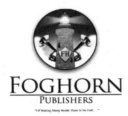

FOGHORN
PUBLISHERS

"Of Making Many Books There Is No End. . ."

Setting Things Straight: Achieving Spectacular Health Without Medical Guesswork, Drastic Dieting and Deadly Drugs

ISBN: 0-9779452-5-1

Printed in the United States of America

Foghorn Publishers
P.O. Box 8286
Manchester, CT 06040-0286
860-216-5622
860-290-8291 fax.
foghornpublisher@aol.com

1 2 3 4 5 6 7 8 9 10 / 09 08 07 06

Disclaimer

————◦•◦————

The information contained in this book is the culmination of 25 years of experience in natural health care, working directly with thousands of patients of all ages. The statements made have not been evaluated by the FDA or the CDC. The opinions expressed are the opinions of the author as well as other qualified natural health experts. The legal climate of our day requires me to tell you that you should not breathe, think, alter your medication, or start any exercise or diet program without first consulting a physician.

The author or the publisher of this material shall have neither liability nor responsibility to any person or entity with respect to any loss, damage or injury caused or alleged to be caused directly by the information contained in this book. The information presented herein is not intended to be a substitute for medical counseling.

The information contained in this book is for informational purposes only and is not intended to diagnose, treat or cure disease or to take the place of care or treatment by a qualified, licensed health care professional. Your results will vary.

For Better Health Naturally
John H. Madeira, D.C

Endorsements

"This book is a bible on natural non-drug health care that will give you amazing wisdom and practical insights that will change your whole life. Corporations and insurance companies who institute Dr. John's ideas and concepts will save millions of dollars! The last chapter on developing your own unique personal wellness plan is a totally revolutionary idea that makes the whole book worth reading."

Robert DeMaria, D.C.
Drugless Health Care Solutions
Author of *How to Stop ADHD in 18 Days* and
Dr. Bob's Trans Fat Survival Guide
Cleveland, OH

SETTING THINGS STRAIGHT

"Dr. John Madeira is a knowledgeable man in the area of natural health. He's tapped into God's laws of health and wellness. You'll be strengthened and enriched as you glean the wisdom of this book."

John Bevere
Author/Speaker, Messenger International
Colorado Springs/United Kingdom/Australia

"Dr John Madeira is a fresh and extremely talented Chiropractor and Natural Health Care Expert who exudes the rare attributes of servant leadership the world desperately needs. His motivation, inspiration, presence and forward thinking, will guide you to newer heights of personal power, wellness mindset and life mastery. All who have been touched by Dr. John have been blessed in their quest for creating an extraordinary quality of life."

Dr. Mike Reid
Fortune Management
Ottawa, Ontario, Canada

Dr. Madeira has added his voice to the revolution in health care and wellness that is transforming our society. Read this book for yourself and your own health. Then apply it's lessons to building a new more sane health care system that values health over disease treatment and patients over procedures and systems.

Guy Reikeman, D.C.
President, Life University
Marietta, GA

Cover to cover this work is Dr. John's tour de force. It's classic Madeira; clear, passionate and convincing. **Setting Things Straight** is nothing short of a deliberate and frontal attack on all that is convenient, mediocre, and status quo in (your) life. I welcome his clarion call to intentional living. He truly believes and lives what he offers his readers. Somehow "Thank you" sounds ridiculously inadequate.

W. Gregory Larsh, Ph.D.
Pastoral Counselor, Educator, Fundraiser

Straightforward, life changing, powerful and insightful... Dr. John has discovered strategic keys to perpetual good health. This book is a *must read* for anyone serious about establishing a lifestyle of good health. His broad perspective and revelation bring a workable plan into focus. His success and expertise in the health field has enabled him to produce a book that will change your life forever!

Dr. Steve Ball
Founder & Pastor, Metropolitan Tabernacle

"Invaluable for anyone wanting to learn from Dr. John Madeira's expertise in natural health care, this book offers a wealth of advice and wisdom essential in the pursuit of health and well being."

Bryan Muir
Washington Capitals

"This book will not just give you great information ...it could save your life."

Bob Harrison
America's Increase Activist

"Extremely educational and thoroughly enjoyable... Dr. Madeira writes in a clear, concise style that is easy to follow and holds the reader's attention. After reading this book, every chiropractor will be more committed, every patient will more readily embrace the chiropractic lifestyle, and every prospective patient will be more willing to fearlessly and whole-heartedly begin care. What an outstanding book! This book is one of the best books written on chiropractic, it is simple, easy to understand and strong in philosophy."

Terry A Rondberg, DC
President, World Chiropractic Alliance

"When you respect the integrity, knowledge and heart of the messenger you can freely and excitedly open up to the message that burns within them. I know John Madeira and have witnessed his lifestyle, practice and family....that's why I know "Setting Things Straight" is a godsend into your life for better health and the education to help bless others".

Dominic Russo
Senior Pastor
Oakland Christian Church
Oakland Twp. Michigan
Russo Family Ministries

"Dr. Madeira deals with many truths about health that are being totally neglected in our lives today. Your life body, soul and spirit will be transformed as you put his principles of health into action in your life."

Mel Weaver
Senior Pastor
Grace Chapel

"I have known Dr. John for many years. I have been privileged to know him as his patient, fellow leader, and friend. The words in this book flow from the burning passion of John's heart: to see people fully enjoying the gift of life. May your body, your mind, and your spirit be refreshed by this liberating book.""

David Hess,
Senior Pastor
Christ Community Church
Camp Hill, PA

Acknowledgements

———— ⊷•⊶ ————

My heartfelt gratitude and appreciation goes out to my wife Karen; you are the love of my life. Thank you for 28 wonderful years of marriage and for your encouragement and support in spreading our message of extraordinary health and well-being to the world. Jonathan and Kayla you are the two best children a father could ask for and the greatest future Chiropractors to be, on the planet. To my Mom and Dad, for your commitment to raising us with Godly values and genuine concern for the interests of others.

Dr. Bob and Deb DeMaria, my mentors and friends who encouraged me to share my message to the world in book form. The team at Madeira Chiropractic who "live it out" everyday and have impacted and saved literally thousands of lives over the last 25 years. Dr. Aaron

D. Lewis, whose wisdom, abilities and talents made this work a reality. To all my partners at Madeira Success Strategies and all Doctors of Chiropractic worldwide for their dedication, perseverance and desire to take the truth about health to the masses. You amaze me and drive me to excel everyday. Thank you! Lastly, to all natural health care providers who work diligently everyday to change people's lives. Your work and your courage have not gone unnoticed.

Table of Contents

———✦———

Introduction xv

Chapter One   The Three Worse Foods to
                Eat and Why 1

Chapter Two   6 Ways To Increase Your Energy by
                100% 21

Chapter Three   Losing Weight Naturally 41

Chapter Four   How To Boost Your Immune
                System 61

Chapter Five   Increasing Your Body's Ability
                to Heal Itself 85

Chapter Six   The Non-Drug Approach to
                Lowering Your Cholesterol 109

Chapter Seven   Diabetes—Prevention and Control . .123

Chapter Eight   Vitamin Supplements—
                Where Do I Begin? 145

Chapter Nine   Conquering Stress the Chiropractic
                Way 163

Chapter Ten   Developing Your Personal
                Wellness Plan—$1 Million Dollar
                Health Habits 179

                Appendix of Chiropractors 193

Introduction

————⇥◆⇤————

With thousands of alternative health and naturopathic remedy books in print, why another one?
It would seem as if the works that already exist
should suffice to adequately cover all of the areas that ail
most people today. Let's face it; you can pretty much
find a book to deal with everything from How To Lose
100 Pounds In One Week, to Having Better Viagra-Free
Sex, to How To Feel Sixteen When You're Sixty. So why
add to the massive collection of well-written works, and
some not so well-written about this often misunderstood
and controversial topic of health?

There are many answers to this question. But lets just
deal with the most obvious one; most books can be quite
confusing. It's not that one book alone is confusing, but
rather when you combine all of them together. Everybody

has vastly different advice to give you. One professional is advising you to eat all of the fat and red meat that your body can consume and guarantees that you'll safely shed pounds. Another expert suggests that you should never eat any fat, and then uses the Bible to add backing to his find.

Some say yes to sugar, others vehemently oppose it. Many diabetic victims and the sugar-conscious tend to use artificial sweeteners as an alternative to the "white stuff," yet some experts claim it can make you senile when taken over a long period of time. I've heard others claim that you can eat like a hog, shun exercise, just think positive thoughts or take a wonder pill and you'll be as healthy as ever. The bottom line is that everybody can't be right, which means that somebody has to be wrong.

But how do we decide on who's right from who's wrong? Or does that really matter at all? We are all on a journey and all at different places on the road to cleaning up our diets and improving our health. That's what this work is all about. It's not so much who's right or who's wrong that we are trying to determine but rather what's right for you. You were created with a very singularly unique quality that makes you very different from anyone else in the world. Much like no two persons share the same social security number, no two persons share the same DNA, making their needs quite different from the next person's.

However, even though we have our differences there are still some things that everybody's body needs no matter who they are or what their special DNA codes are. I call these things absolutes. For example everybody needs air without which you will die. People need water intake in order for their internal organs to work optimally. Whether it's spring water, distilled water, or tap water may not be as important as the fact that you are actually taking in water. The need for water and air are absolutes that most people know and have come to accept, whether or not they choose to admit it.

There are other absolutes that may not be as well known as those are. Because they are not as commonly understood does not mean that they have any less authenticity. One such absolute that is the thread that weaves all good health tightly together is having a healthy spine. Without a healthy, well-aligned spine, and healthy nerve supply getting to all parts of your body, it really does not matter how many of the other areas you have in proper position. Lack of awareness of proper spinal care, has become a universal concern at this point in time. Improper alignment of the body, especially the spine and its consequential effects on proper nerve supply will invariably cause negative reactions to occur in your body affecting your overall health.

But while there are what I call absolutes, (which we'll discuss in far greater detail throughout this book), there are also things that can easily be contested and even totally refuted with very little hard proof. For example, when I ask most people in my seminars and workshops the simple question, "Does prescription medication heal people or even make people healthier?" Most respond with a pretty firm, "no." People are not stupid, and this I know particularly when they continue to give the right answers about their health and how vastly limited prescription medication has been, in their personal experiences.

The truth is you do not have to get sick, suffer or succumb to disease.

Nonetheless, much like Pavlov's dog salivating at the sound of the ringing bell, many people cannot seem to break the futile habit of taking drugs though they know that it's not working for them. Some habits tend to be harder to break than others and the "drug" habit fueled by billions of dollars of medical propaganda and marketing seems to have always been on the top of the list.

Another long accepted notion that can be refuted is that sickness and disease are inevitable, as we get older. I'll admit that when you look around that statement seems to be pretty reasonable. But remember, looks can be very deceiving. The truth is you do not have to get sick, suffer or succumb to disease. If you make good choices you can live a long, healthy, drug-free life and I will show you how.

While most people don't know that they have other options and real alternatives to healthcare as we have come to know it, it is my objective to inform you of those options while *setting things straight.* One option in particular is making sense of all the drug company hype, medical brainwashing, fear factors and misinformation that you have been taught to believe to be true, which in fact are not true at all.

In *Setting Things Straight: Achieving Spectacular Health Without Medical Guesswork, Drastic Dieting and Deadly Drugs,* I am going to show you how to get past your pain, prevent sickness and disease, and have the best health that you can possibly have. Remember that there are some things that are absolutes and other areas that are shaded, or worse yet outright untrue. You'll need to know which is which if you're going to experience an optimal quality of life and health.

Using my thirty-three years experience in natural health care combined with the borrowed knowledge of what I believe are some of the best written works on the subject of healthcare. I intend to inspire you to plot out your own personal wellness master plan, one that works best for your lifestyle, your body and where you presently are on your journey. If you experience perfect health after reading and applying this work I will be sincerely grateful. However, perfection is not really my immediate goal for you but rather improvement.

SETTING THINGS STRAIGHT

If you can use any of the information presented in this work and be able to honestly say that it has helped you to improve in one or more areas of your life, then I've successfully accomplished my goal. Furthermore if you from now on will vow to use your own heart and mind to make quality decisions that you intuitively know are best for your overall health and be able to ask more intelligent questions, then I'll know without any doubt that I've not only reached my desired goal but that I have also helped you to *set things straight* in the process.

Every valley shall be filled in, every mountain and hill made low. The crooked roads shall become straight, the rough ways smooth. Luke 3:5

—John H. Madeira, D.C.
Hershey, PA

CHAPTER ONE

The Three Worse Foods To Eat And Why

A story is told about a turkey farmer who was taking a walk one day and found an eagle's egg. He thought it was a turkey egg so he threw it into his turkey pen. The egg later hatched and the eagle began to grow up around turkeys. So the eagle grew up thinking in his mind that he was a turkey and spent his entire life scratching and pecking at the ground. One day when the eagle was very old he spotted a beautiful bird soaring and diving among the clouds. When he inquired of his turkey friend what kind of bird it actually was, he replied "Oh that is an eagle, the king of the sky. But don't pay any mind to him.

Eagles were meant to fly and to soar. We were born to walk and peck." And so the eagle that thought he was a bona fide turkey went back to walking and pecking. The moral of the story is not to walk and peck when you were created to soar. If you want to start acting like an eagle you have to stop thinking like a turkey. Unfortunately many of the things that we have been taught or lead to believe about health are now known to not be true. It is my goal to help you to think like an eagle when it comes to you and your family's health and overall well-being. That will mean that you will have to become more open to some ideas that may soar far above the ideals that you've been taught over the years.

Living a healthy life and making healthy choices should not be drudgery and burdensome, but rather an enjoyable experience that you look forward to practicing every day. I like the concept of keeping things simple, as simple as possible. So I've made it easy for you in this chapter to avoid what I believe are the three most potentially harmful foods, and I'll give you reasons why you should do so.

Some authors, (and of course it's their prerogative), give you such a long list of do's and don'ts that unless you're Albert Einstein or Professor Stephen W. Hawking, you won't remember one tenth of the list, of what you should from what you should not eat. The bottom line is that long lists of "what not to eat" only leads to, frustration, starvation and too often out-of-control binging. In all reality you have to eat to live. Yet there are some things that are harmful if you consume too much of them, I realize that. But trying to talk you out of eating your grandmother's favorite dish, or Thanksgiving dinner is probably not going to work. So I've adopted a fresher approach.

While there are plenty of killer foods in our fast-paced, fast food society, I've chosen to deal with the ones that'll kill you quickest. If you can master the art of avoiding just these three food types, you may not necessarily win the Boston Marathon, but you will be on the road to better health than you've ever experienced before and on your way to creating a healthier future for yourself. I've read lists in books, listing twenty, thirty, and often more than fifty foods that are strictly prohibited. After reading the list I wondered to myself if there were any foods left for me to eat at all except for kale and turnip greens, whatever they are. Let's keep this real. Eating the right foods play a very important role in your overall health, but just eating from the right food groups is no guarantee of great and vibrant health just by itself.

There are other things that play a very important role such as regular exercise, proper sleep, decreasing your stress levels, appropriate water intake, and also having a healthy spine. It's everything working synergistically with each other that spawns great health in your body, not one magical thing alone. So you may eat all the right foods yet never exercise your body or get any physical activity leaving a gaping hole for sickness to enter your life. Your blood has to move throughout your body to properly oxygenate and nourish your cells and tissues. Exercise stimulates blood flow, improves digestion and maintains the flexibility of your joints.

Okay then, you exercise pretty regularly but you eat things that are loaded with bad fats. In that case it would probably be better if you did not exercise at all, seeing that your blood stream is clogged with unhealthy fats, which blocks healthy flow and potentially leads to fatal clotting. Perhaps you may be like the millions of unaware health seekers, who sincerely do all of the above on the list of daily healthy habits, yet omit proper spinal care. That may be one of the most frustrating scenarios. You actually have a healthy body in one sense but are still developing "behind the scenes" problems because your spine, which is your lifeline, is not properly aligned, causing future problems that won't rear their ugly heads for years to come.

So this work is not about just eating right or exercising, or piling up on vitamins. It's your step-by-step guide to give you small things to do that will all eventually add up to great health. What's the incentive? Everybody wants an incentive in life. Why should you give up this or start doing that, just because I say so? You shouldn't. You should only do what I suggest because you believe deep down within that you are going to receive a corresponding benefit in exchange.

Unless you are totally deranged, I'd suspect that you probably want to live as long as you can. I know that I do want to live long, as long as I am well and able to enjoy my life. Making these choices, and implementing these small steps, little by little, will help you to do just that. But why do you want to live longer? Hopefully, you have purpose and destiny on your life. I trust that you have a driving force within you wanting to do more than you've ever done before, endeavoring to leave this world a better place because you've been here. I believe that because you are actually reading this book that you are on a higher thinking level than more than eighty percent of the world's population.

You are reading this book simply because you do give a care. And deep within, you care about making a difference in the lives of other people. If those are not enough motivations to begin to adopt new habits, then how about his one—*you will simply feel great.* Nothing in life should matter more to your physical body than feeling as good as you possibly can. If you don't consider that enough motivation, visit the hospital, or convalescent home in your area, and ask the patients if feeling great once again is a high or low priority to them? You may want to take the afternoon off, because I'm sure they'll have a whole lot to tell you.

So many people take healthy living for granted or they simply *hope* they will live long and healthy. I do not believe that you are one of those people. I believe you really want to feel great all of the time and are interested in planting seeds today that will produce long term fruit of wholeness and health in your life . But don't just consider a healthier way of life, because you've been forced to through some type of emergency circumstance. Don't wait for a negative report from your medical doctor or for an accident to begin this journey.

If you are already there, that's fine. The advice I will be giving you is good for both those who are desperate to get their health back as well as for those of you who want to fly with the eagles your whole life through. Don't wait for bad news. You are your own anchorperson and you get the privilege of forecasting your own future, your effectiveness, your contributions to life, and your health. You are in control, what's the forecast for today? Before you answer that, let's deal with some things that we don't ever want to see in the forecast anymore.

The Low Down On Sugar

Of the deadliest foods in the history of mankind, sugar is arguably the worst and perhaps the deadliest food available for human consumption. Let me explain. When I speak of sugar, I am not talking about natural sweeteners such as honey, date sugar, real maple syrup or stevia natural sweeteners. I am talking about the white stuff—processed bleached sugar that is sold in five to ten

pound bags in your local grocery store, that are affecting billions of sweet tooth consumers worldwide.

The very process of making sugar into the form that
we've come to accept as normal is pretty repulsive. But
before we deal with that, lets talk about where sugar
comes from. First, sugar is made from one of two
sources, the sugar cane, a very tall grass, with large
stems, resembling a bamboo plant, that grow mostly in
tropical regions. Sugar cane sugar accounts for seventy
percent of the world's production of sugar. The remain-
ing thirty percent comes from the sugar beet, which is a
root crop that looks very much like the a parsnip, grown
mostly in the north under more moderate temperatures.

More than 120 countries contribute in the overall production of sugar. The United States alone produces nearly 7
million tons annually. How is it made? The first stage of processing sugar is called affination. In this stage the raw sugar
is softened and then the layer of mother liquor around the
crystals is removed. The sugar then goes through a process
of carbonation where the solids, or clumps of sugar, which
make up the liquor are removed. After this is done the sugar
liquor is ready for de-colorization where ions remove the
color from and bleach the sugar.

Then finally they boil water until it's just optimal for
sugar crystals to grow. Once the sugar crystals have
grown, the mixture is then spun around until they are
separated out. They are then hot-air dried and ready for

packaging. It doesn't really sound like all that bad of a process, right? I forgot to mention that the entire process of separation, breaking down the molecules, and discoloring the grains, is all done with the use of noxious chemicals that are extremely harmful to your body.

In fact, the process is so harmful that it has been proven that white refined sugar has been a leading cause of the majority of the major diseases with which people suffer everyday. You probably think that you don't consume that much sugar, but you'd be surprised. The average person consumes about their body weight in sugar per year, plus an additional 20 pounds in corn syrup.

Sugar is in nearly everything that we eat. It's in alcohol, ketchup, candy, soda, desserts, fruit juices, wine, beer, bread, most processed foods, and the list could continue on and on. Even if you throw away all the white sugar in your house, (and I suggest that you do) and never buy it again, chances are highly probable that you will still consume sugar, especially if you ever order food from a restaurant or fast food joint. Food manufacturers sneak it into foods all the time without our knowledge.

"According to the World Health Organization, no more than 10 percent of calories should come from added sweeteners. This advice is in line with the long-standing recommendations of the U.S. Department of Agriculture food pyramid, called for a maximum of 12 teaspoons of sugar (48 grams) in a 2,200-

calorie diet, which translates to roughly 9 percent of daily calories." [1]

These recommendations are extremely high in my opinion. Let me explain. What does sugar actually do to the body? The main problem is that sugar puts a strain on the immune system, the system that protects the body from getting sick or developing disease. Intake of sugar causes the pancreas to secrete abnormal amounts of insulin, which is required to break the sugar down. Insulin causes the cells in the body to store the sugar in the form of fat. Yep, now you know why America is so fat. High sugar consumption is making us the fattest nation on earth and raising Diabetes and it's complications to epidemic proportions.

In addition after the sugar has been metabolized, the insulin still remains in the blood. And when insulin stays in the blood past its expiration time, it hinders the release of growth hormones in the pituitary gland. So children that eat large amounts of sugar can encounter growth hormone deficiency.

The body does not recognize white sugar as a real food, but rather treats it as if it is a poison in the system, (particularly since it has heavy-duty chemicals in it) that need to be expelled from the body.

---

1. Source: http://www.ahealthyme.com/topic/toomuchsugar

SETTING THINGS STRAIGHT

The problem with sugar is that it causes enormous amounts of health problems and is the culprit in many major diseases. Joseph Mercola, D.O. author of *Dr. Mercola's Total Health Program* and his latest book, *Sweet Deception: Why Splenda®, Nutrasweet®, and the FDA May Be Hazardous To Your Health*, believes that not only is sugar ruining people's health but that the alternative artificial sweeteners approved by the FDA are far more deadly than sugar.

On his website, he lists *76 Ways Sugar Can Ruin Your Health*, which was contributed by Nancy Appleton author of Lick the Sugar Habit Sugar Counter. Here are just a few of the ways that I thought would be most interesting for you to know.

1. *Sugar can suppress your immune system and impair your defenses against infectious disease.*

2. *Sugar can produce a significant rise in total cholesterol, triglycerides and bad cholesterol and a decrease in good cholesterol.*

3. *Sugar feeds cancer cells and has been connected with the development of cancer of the breast, ovaries, prostate, rectum, pancreas, biliary tract, lung, gallbladder and stomach.*

4. *Sugar can increase fasting levels of glucose and can cause hypoglycemia.*

5. *Sugar can weaken eyesight.*

6. *Sugar can cause premature aging.*

7. *Sugar contributes to obesity.*

8. *Sugar can cause autoimmune diseases such as: arthritis, asthma, multiple sclerosis.*

9. *Sugar can cause toxemia during pregnancy.*

10. *Sugar can contribute to eczema in children.*

11. *Sugar intake is higher in people with Parkinson's disease.*

12. *Sugar can increase your risk of Alzheimer's disease.*

13. *Sugar can cause headaches, including migraines.*

14. *Sugar can increase your risk of gout.*

15. *High sugar intake can cause epileptic seizures.*

And I'll add one final thought to this abridged list; sugar is addictive. That is why the sugar habit is so hard to kick, and why we crave it so strongly. In addition to the physical problems that sugar can induce, studies have shown that sugar causes social and behavioral problems also. Here are some of the finds:

Sugar consumption in the USA is so high that it has also caused a social problem through its deleterious

SETTING THINGS STRAIGHT

effects on behavior, especially in children, who are displaying increasingly severe behavioral disorders and learning disabilities.

In a recent study conducted by Dr. C. Keith Connors of the Children's Hospital in Washington, DC, a 'deadly' link was established between the consumption of sugar with carbohydrates (such as breakfast cereal, cake, and biscuits) and violent behavior, hypertension, and learning impediments.

In other studies, chronic violence in prisons was remarkably reduced simply by eliminating refined sugar and starch from prison diets. Singapore in 1991 banned sugary soft drink sales from all schools and youth centers, citing the danger that sugar poses to the mental and physical health of children.[2]

Most people were only taught about the affects that sugar has on your overall dental health. But as you have read, its harmful ramifications go far beyond that beautiful smile of yours. Plainly stated, sugar is the precursor to death. It is poison and should not be consumed, not even in low dosages. Okay, you are wondering, "What if I eat sugar in moderation, that'll be fine, right? Wrong! How small of a dose of cocaine or heroin would you give your child? Hopefully you answered, none. The point is that poison is not food and should have never been categorized

---

2. Source: http://www.hps-online.com (Helping People Survive)

with whole foods to begin with. Keep sugar in its rightful place, away from your body.

What's the Big Deal About Trans Fats and What are They?

The phrase "trans fat" is not quite yet a household name, but it soon will be. Trans fats are actually common cooking oils that have been chemically modified to add shelf life and added texture to commercially manufactured food products. Trans fats are most often labeled as *partially hydrogenated oil.* They are easily spotted on food labels so keep a constant lookout for them. They are nasty and found commonly in peanut butter, margarine, butter replacements, processed cheeses, crackers, cookies, cupcakes, frequently in potato chips and often in pretzels. The absolute worst offender is French fries bought at fast food restaurants. Sorry! One author compared fast food French fries to cigarettes in terms of their deleterious effects on the body.

It has been proven that transitional fats have a devastating effect on the body. The problem is that trans fats cannot be properly digested like natural cooking oils. It's a complicated process to explain but suffice it to say that the abnormal breakdown of these unhealthy chemically modified oils cause pain and inflammation in the body. Some experts believe that they cause cancer and it is proven that they increase cholesterol levels, raising so-called bad cholesterol and lowering good cholesterol.

Most companies that produce foods with transitional fats in their products tend to downplay the magnitude of its potential harmfulness, since the general public is just not educated to the overall meaning of transitional fat as of yet.

When asked by the big food producers what is transitional fat, they've all come up with a very nice sounding coined response that makes them look like really responsible companies with your health and well being on the top of their priority list.

They'll say:

Trans fats are "transitional fats" between saturated and unsaturated, and can be present in hydrogenated oils and also, to a much smaller degree, in animal products such as meat and dairy products. We are currently analyzing all of our products for trans fat in anticipation of new labeling rules, which will require our products to label trans fat by the year 2006.

Then they end by saying:

Most or many of our products are Trans-fat free.

Sounds good right! But it's just not true. According to Dr. Robert DeMaria, author of *Dr. Bob's Trans Fat Survival Guide: Why No Fat, Low Fat, Trans Fat Is Killing You!,* Trans Fat is America's most dangerous fat. Trans Fat clearly contributes to heart disease but it is something that is relatively new to the consumer environment. Trans Fat alters cell membrane structure. It causes pain and inflammation.

He states also that nearly every food that you can purchase at a fast food restaurant has Trans Fat and public school lunch menus are loaded with Trans Fats. It is the precursor to many problems such as childhood obesity and Attention Deficit Disorder.

To find out more about trans fat read: *Dr. Bob's Trans Fat Survival Guide: Why No Fat, Low Fat, Trans Fat Is Killing You!* —Dr Bob DeMaria.

Soda—America's Number One Health Drink?

I always give people the benefit of the doubt. It's just the way I'm wired. So I sincerely believe people intuitively already know that soda is not good for them, yet they still choose to drink it. I realize that we have already dealt with the sugar issue, and you are probably wondering why mention soda, especially since it contains so much sugar? Well one reason is that soda is one of the most highly consumed foods on the market. And young children and teenagers may consume as much or more soda than adults do.

...the average 13-18 year old boy consumes nearly 24 ounces of soda a day.

For example, the average 13-18 year old boy consumes nearly 24 ounces of soda a day. That's two standard-sized soda cans. A 12-ounce can of soda contains nine teaspoons of sugar. One teaspoon of sugar contains about 16 calories. That's a whopping 288 calories in just soda alone, not including the high calories in the snacks, and junk food, that the soda was used to wash down. That may not sound like much to you, but not only do calories add up quickly, both you and I know that most teenagers go far beyond the estimated averages with nearly everything. So those figures are quite conservative.

What bothers me most is that billions of advertising dollars are spent annually from major soda corporations with the intention of targeting youth and small children. It's not much different than the drug dealer on the street corner targeting his or her target market, knowing that once their hooked they'll be clients for life, or should I say until death. I believe that everyone should have a fair shake when it comes to earning an honest living. But these companies are going too far. Soda is the number one cause of fatness in America and is the reason for the high rise in juvenile Diabetes.

My problem is not so much the marketing or the propaganda that usually accompanies the ads but rather the blatant lies that some of them tell or pay others to tell which totally confuses and tricks people into innocently buying into a false notion. Michael F. Jacobson Ph.D. states from an advertisement in his book, *Liquid Candy: How Soft Drinks are Harming American's Health,*

> *The soft drink industry has consistently portrayed its products as being positively healthful, saying*

they are 90 percent water and contain sugars found in nature. A poster that the National Soft Drink Association (now the American Beverage Association) once provided to teachers stated: "As refreshing sources of needed liquids and energy, soft drinks represent a positive addition to a well-balanced diet....These same three sugars also occur naturally, for example, in fruits....In your body it makes no difference whether the sugar is from a soft drink or a peach."

Currently, in a desperate attempt to link soft drinks to good health, the industry emphasizes that soda contains water, an essential nutrient: "Drink plenty of fluids: consume at least eight glasses of fluids daily, even more when you exercise. A variety of beverages, including soft drinks, can contribute to proper hydration." A similar claim was made in 1998 by M. Douglas Ivester, then Coca-Cola's chairman and CEO, when he defended the marketing of soft drinks in Africa. He said, "Actually, our product is quite healthy. Fluid replenishment is a key to health....Coca-Cola does a great service because it encourages people to take in more and more liquids."

Lies, lies, lies! Can you believe that anyone would try to compare the contents of soda to the mineral rich, vitamin-filled fibrous contents in fruits, or the life-sustaining attributes of water? The real truth is that soda has no nutritional value whatsoever. Yes it contains 90 percent water, but the water that it contains is normally not natural spring water neither is it distilled drinking water. Of course, you would never know the difference anyway since it's loaded down with so much sugar, coloring and chemicals you can't even begin to pronounce. You couldn't distinguish whether it was fresh water or toilet water if you wanted to.

Here is something more to think about. I believe that the reason we enjoy soda is the bubbles not the taste. The carbonation is stimulating to our mouths. We don't ever drink flat soda, do we? Remove the carbonation and we have a big fat zero in the taste department. Try to get your kids to drink old soda. *Ain't going to happen!* If you think about it, soda really doesn't taste very good. It's just cold and it sizzles.

If you want to know the truth, here it is. Rather than being a health drink with natural fruit and quality drinking water, soda consumption is directly connected to:

- Obesity
- Bone Deterioration
- Osteoporosis
- Tooth Decay
- Heart Disease
- Kidney Stone and Renal Failure
- Mood swings

- Anxiety and Restlessness

And that's just a small list. My job here is not to demonize food or pull scare tactics on you. No, my job is very clearly to help you to think. You need to think for yourself. But this time you need to be able to think with some factual information, not with the lies they've told you. I want to help you take back control, total control over your body, and the money hungry vultures that will lie to your face, just to create the sale. In some ways the food industry has behaved like the tobacco industry putting profits ahead of conscious.

One of the things that many people believe is that drinking diet soda has a less harmful affect on your body. That's not true. For the most part people tend to drink diet sodas to be more mindful of their weight. According to eight years of information collected by Sharon P. Fowler, MPH, and colleagues at the University of Texas, diet drinks may actually cause you to gain weight rather than aid in weight loss. Fowler and her team of researchers were not a bit surprised about the fact that soda increases obesity. What was surprising was that the people drinking diet soft drinks had a higher risk of obesity than those that drank regular soda. Whether diet or straight, soda is just not a healthy choice, no matter what flavor it may come in.

You do have options, and you have the right to exercise those options. One of your rights is the right to good health. So as a health professional I strongly believe that it is my obligation to inform you when any concerted conspiratorial effort is trying to steal your most precious asset from you. The time to take back your health is NOW!

I would like to make one last comment on another up and coming popular beverage. One very popular sports-related drink (to remain nameless) is fast, becoming thought of as a healthier alternative to soda but could not be farther from the truth. These drinks popularized as the new drink of choice for athletes to replace electrolytes are full of artificial food dyes, chemicals, sugar and salt. Their strongly implied health benefits are staggeringly, outweighed by their detrimental ingredients. Use your common sense and don't fall for the lie. Nothing is ever going to be better for hydration than good old-fashioned water.

CHAPTER TWO

6 Ways To Increase Your Energy By 100%

One of the things that I have noticed over the many years in my practice is the growing number of fatigued and lethargic people that I come face to face with on a regular basis. This seems to be increasingly more the rule than the exception. Before you automatically assume that I am referring to older aged people, think again. I find more and more young people, and young adults lacking the energy that is more commonly associated with youthfulness. Actually, I tend to see middle-aged adults and often seniors, participating in sports and other activities that you would normally expect younger people to participate in. Let me explain.

I know guys and gals in their fifties, sixties, and seventies, that still go skiing, and I don't mean on the bunny slopes. Many of these people play basketball, ride bicycles cross country, run marathons, play tennis, swim two to three miles each day, and some even go mountain climbing. One of my 70 plus year old patients plays tennis regularly and drives not rides a Harley Davidson. Cool! The point that I want you to understand is that having the kind of energy that you truly desire is not a matter of age, but it is rather a matter of choice.

And with that choice there are some things that you can do right now, to tap into the wellspring of energy lying dormant in you. I've provided you with six different options to pursue to get your energy back. Eventually I recommend that you address each area. But more realistically I am simply trying to get you to do one maybe even two out of the six things listed here. Remember, this book is not about finding ways to overwhelm you. It's about providing simple workable alternatives that you choose. Each thing that you add will in time have a compounded affect on your life, level of wellness and your overall productivity.

The list of the ways that you can increase your energy is not necessarily in a sequential order. You choose which of the things works best for you right now. Whatever area you believe that you can improve on most is the area that you should begin exploring. You know what's right for your body better than anyone else; I am simply here to remind you.

Improve Your Diet!

American trends have influenced the entire world. From New Orleans Jazz Music, Elvis Presley's signature Memphis styled Rock & Roll, to New York styled clothing, and East and West Coast rap beats, to Oprah Winfrey's prime time broadcasting, to Philly Cheese Steaks: you can pretty much see characteristics of American culture in nearly every major city in the world. Some of our influences are good and others are not good at all. One such negative influence is our dietary habits and the proliferation of fast food joints on nearly every part of the globe. Most people are totally oblivious to the major health hazards of fast food.

Just as innocently as a baby reaches for a sharp object and puts it into her mouth, or a toddler sticks a paper clip into an electrical wall outlet, millions of people run to buy food in a hurry from these places, every single day, not even once considering the danger involved. Let's just use some common sense for a moment. If you are thirty years old or older it is pretty safe to say that you have probably witnessed someone cooking a meal in the kitchen. Let's say that the person who you were watching cook was your mother, aunt, or grandmother, possibly your dad or granddad.

For the sake of the illustration let's also say they were cooking a piece of beef or possibly a hamburger. How long did it take to cook? Two minutes, three or four, or maybe try about twenty to thirty minutes to cook a piece of ground beef thoroughly. Now I have not even added in the time that it took for preparation. Old-fashioned burgers were kneaded like dough, massaging all of the ingredients and seasonings into the beef. Some added ingredients were pieces of bread, onions, chopped peppers, and of course salt and black pepper. After that, the mix would get carefully shaped into thick circular burgers, and then they were ready to be cooked.

So to make about four or five burgers could have easily taken forty-five minutes considering all the preparation involved. Seems like too much time to wait? Actually it is not. That is the amount of time that is really needed to cook a piece of fresh meat safely. But those days seem to be long forgotten now. And that's one reason why people are more sick than ever. How long does it take for you to get a burger from McDonald's, Wendy's, or Burger King? I realize that they require less preparation time since they don't add in the fresh onions and peppers into the actual burger. They put them on the outside, it's much quicker and everybody doesn't like the same things.

But how long does it take? Five minutes, four, try again. It takes less than two minutes from the time you order to the time that your burger is actually bagged and given to you with a smile. That's a scary thing. I've already asked you to use your common sense, so how in the world can any healthy food be prepared in less than two minutes. Even a tossed salad requires more time than that. The truth of the matter is that fast preparation is really no preparation at all. That may sound strange at first, but it's true. The reason why they can make you a burger that fast, is because their patties come already prepared shrink wrapped and ready to fry.

At the break of the century hamburgers were considered to be food for the poor, and were usually only found at carnivals, circuses, and from street vendors. But with the popularization of fast food, the burger has become far more conventional, socially acceptable, and more lethal. I believe the fast food habit is the beginning of bad eating habits and bad health in children. Burgers were not necessarily health food when momma cooked them, but now there is no argument at all, they work against good health. And many of the problems, which our children suffer from, may be connected to their diet, a diet of convenience, especially obesity and behavioral problems.

Although I am not vouching for high intake of red meat, I am saying that when mother cooked your meat you at least knew what it was. Today, you don't know what's in the food. Well perhaps you do but just don't want to accept it. Some of what's in our children's lunch provided by the public school system is pretty disgusting. In his book *Fast Food Nation: The Dark Side of the All American Meal*, Eric Schlosser says:

> *Throughout the 1980s and 1990s, the USDA chose meat suppliers for its National School Lunch Program on the basis of the lowest price, without imposing additional food safety requirements. The cheapest ground beef was not only the most likely to be contaminated with pathogens, but also the most likely to contain pieces of spinal cord, bone, and gristle left behind by Automated Meat Recovery Systems (contraptions that squeeze the last shreds of meat off bones).*
>
> *A 1983 investigation by NBC News said that the Cattle King Packing Company—at the time, the USDA's largest supplier of ground beef for school lunches and a supplier to Wendy's—routinely processed cattle that were already dead before arriving at the plant, hid diseased cattle from inspectors, and mixed rotten meat that had been returned by customers into packages of hamburger meat. Cattle King's facilities were infested with rats and cockroaches. (218)*

I know that is pretty gross but it's quite unfortunate that things are not the same as they used to be. But since you know that, make a quality decision to kick the fast food habit all together. Although I've used ground beef as my example, I could have just as easily used chicken, particularly as it relates to fast food restaurants. It has been a generally accepted thought by health practitioners for years that chicken is a far better and healthier choice than beef. Perhaps that may be true when you compare chicken to beef rather than chicken parts to beef parts.

Predominantly, all of the ingredients headed for the fast food chains are inferior ingredients and all share a very similar alluring yet sickening quality to them. Chicken parts ground up and smashed together into a nugget then breaded and deep-fried in bad oil or hanging out inside of a taco are still both highly processed meats and generally have little nutritional value.

Predominantly, all of the ingredients headed for the fast food chains are inferior ingredients and all share a very similar alluring yet sickening quality to them.

All of these life-taking foods hinder your energy in the process by slowly wearing you down. As much as you possibly can, eat whole foods. What I mean by whole foods are foods that come from the earth. Increase your vegetable and fruit intake. Choose food from a farm over food from a factory. If you are going to eat meat at least know where it comes from.

Eating more vegetables and fresh fruit not canned, will increase the fiber in your diet. These foods actually add

Choose food from a farm over food from a factory.

⌒

energy to you since they have lots of vitamins and minerals that your body needs. The fiber actually helps your digestion tremendously and moves poisons and toxins through your bowels faster. Backup and reabsorption of toxins and waste products of digestion in your bowels can dramatically lower your energy levels.

You may not like the taste of anything natural for awhile especially if you have become addicted to a fast food diet because it is loaded with salt and sometimes sugar. The purpose of that is to keep you coming back for more. Food companies know what drives us. We have already established that sugar, trans fats and soda are the three worst foods we can eat. They steal energy by taxing your liver, robbing the body of vital vitamins and minerals and sending your blood sugar levels on a roller coaster ride.

What I ask, is that you start where you are. Choose a healthy food that you've not been accustomed to eating; and add it into your daily eating plan. Take one thing candy bars and replace it with something healthier.

If you are considering dieting, don't starve yourself. Some diets recommend that you eat only one meal a day. Actually you'll be hungrier and be far more prone to binge when you follow such a plan. I suggest that you eat smaller controlled portions more often. Your body needs food to create energy. And the more that you feed your body (moderately), the less your body will actually have to borrow from you to create energy leaving you tired and feeling worn out. Making wiser food choices will increase your energy.

Exercise More Regularly

Don't get scared; I'm not going to sign you up for the next marathon or Iron Man triathlon. What I will suggest is that you begin to increase your physical activity. It may be as simple as taking a walk around the block or slipping in an exercise DVD and following the instructions. Often, people believe that in order for you to get more exercise that you've got to join a gym and workout three to five times a week. That is great for the person whose schedule is conducive for that kind of regimen. But if you can't make it to the gym there are still plenty of things that you can do to work your body out. It can be as easy as starting a walking program 20 minutes everyday at lunchtime or taking your dog for walks. It will be good for Rover also.

Fitness trainer Denise Austin actually shows on her television program a myriad of ways that you can get a complete workout using a mop stick. She actually proved that you could use a mop stick and work the majority of your major muscles. Back in my high school football days we would train by running up and down the school stairwells. That helped to build our calves and gave us a pretty major cardiovascular workout, at the same time. If you have stairs in your house, or if you live in an apartment building, or on the second floor or higher, you can simply walk up and down the stairs more than normal and get a pretty serious workout. It really doesn't have to be hard.

There are many Amish people in Lancaster, Pennsylvania, about an hour's drive from my clinic. I go there to an Amish farm every week to adjust my patients. One of the amazing things is that these precious people do not go to the gym, they don't have workout facilities in their homes, and they don't have electricity, televisions or DVD players, which means they cannot listen to Denise Austin or Billy Blanks Tae Bo tapes. However, these Amish brethren are some of my most healthy patients. While they may not receive the kind of exercise that we've come to label as conventional exercise, they get more exercise than the faithful fitness freaks in the gym three and four times each week pumping iron.

Everyday, the Amish people use their bodies all day, to plant food in their gardens, to make and repair their own clothing, to harvest their crops, and to cultivate the ground for new crops. When they want milk, they don't drive to the store and buy milk like you and I would. They instead milk the cows. They also shovel the manure. What I've named is just a small portion of the many activities that they perform on any given day. All of these exercises require physical strength and aptitude. And they work like this all of the time. For them, it is a lifestyle.

They do it without knowing that they are actually doing it. That has to be one of the greatest secrets to exercise. Find something involving physical activity that you either love to do or have to do, either works. And simply increase your involvement in that task. Your blood has tremendous healing properties within it and carries life-giving nutrition and oxygen. However, if it is not flowing properly

One of the mysteries of the human body is that you must give energy to get energy back.

because of a lack of physical activity and body movement then your body won't heal normally, leaving you in pain, low on power and wanting to go to sleep simply to escape the pain.

The old adage is still true. Whatever you give will come back to you. If you give love you'll receive love. When you give money generously you can surely expect it to come back to you with interest. And when you exert energy, although you may feel tired at first, new energy is looking to replenish the old energy used. That's just the way the body works. God designed the body to heal itself. One of the mysteries of the human body is that you must give energy to get energy back.

Improve Your Brain/Body Connections by Seeing Your Chiropractor

Our body is actually made up of trillions of cells that make up our tissues and organs. Those cells are all connected directly to our brains by way of a vast network of nerve pathways known as our nerve system. Your brain is very much like your very own PC or personal computer, that directs and controls every function in your body by sending messages down your spinal cord. Nerve messages flow from the brain down the nerves of the spinal cord, out small openings between your spinal bones and then to your organs and body tissues.

Literally every cell is in direct or indirect communication with the brain at all times. Nerve messages travel over the nerves like electricity flows through a copper wire and they control your heart beat, your blood pressure, digestion, immune system strength, liver and kidney function, blood cell production, body temperature regulation and body movements just to name a few. Volumes of research and scientific books have been written trying to describe what we know about the functions of the nerve system and our understanding is still very limited. But what we do know is that misalignments of the spinal bones inhibits the proper flow of the nerve messages and interfere with the body's ability to heal itself and to keep itself working properly. Chiropractors call these misalignments 'subluxations' which means minor dislocation of a spinal bone. While that may sound painful most often it is not. In fact most people have several of them in their spine and are completely unaware that they are secretly causing problems elsewhere in their body.

Subluxations short circuit the brain/body connections. Misalignment of the spinal bones is most commonly caused by incidents such as birth trauma, slips and falls, car accidents, talking repeatedly on the phone while it is kinked under your shoulder, sleeping on a bad mattress or pillow, falling asleep on the couch watching TV, sports impacts and childhood falls. Research has shown that most of us have had at least one subluxation before the age of two. What that means is that many of us, in fact most, have brain/body connection problems. These misalignments in the spine are the root cause of many of the unwanted conditions that people suffer from every day.

> *Your spine is the switchboard of the body.*

Your spine is the switchboard of the body. It consists of twenty four bones called vertebrae which are supposed to be in proper alignment for you to feel your best and for your body to work at its best. Misalignments rob the body of needed energy big time and literally cause all kinds of health problems such as allergies, asthma, sinusitis, ear infections in children, stress and migraines headaches, chronic fatigue syndrome, low energy, neck and back pain and curvature of the spine to name just a few problems Chiropractors routinely help.

Chiropractors are to the spine what Orthodontists are to teeth. We are rigorously trained for eight years to evaluate the health and alignment of the spine and its impact on the rest of the body. The treatment delivered by Chiropractors, called a chiropractic adjustment is a very safe and painless procedure that won't harm even the spine of a tiny infant. Chiropractic adjustments restore the normal nerve flow from the brain to the body and back. In order for your energy to be strong and for you to feel and function at your best it is imperative that your spine be checked and adjusted to remove subluxations on a regular basis.

Get More Sleep

Another reason why you are tired is that you are not getting enough sleep. I know you went to sleep last night and woke up this morning, but that is not what I am talking about. I mean proper rest, seven to eight hours of uninterrupted sleep. Most people are far too busy, or at least believe they are, and factor out the possibility of having regular healthy sleep patterns. They mistakenly believe that they can get by on 5 or 6 hours of rest a night. This is a false belief. Not only does that create what sleep experts call a sleep deficit but it strains our immune resistance. I almost never get sick (because I do all of the things I am recommending to you) but when I do it is almost always because of a lack of consistent sleep over a several day period of time. Sleep recharges and refreshes your body and helps keep your immune system strong.

When you sleep at night, you give the body the chance to rejuvenate itself and prepare for the realities of a brand new day. Imagine what would happen if you continued to use your cell phone, yet the battery was signaling the low battery warning sign? No matter how important your conversation was it would be interrupted because the battery will shut off power to the phone until it gets recharged. It can only work for so long. We often work past our body's function-ability levels, and though

While you sleep your blood is actually being cleansed and your body rebuilds, repairs and rejuvenates itself.

our body is saying, "quit, end for the day," we continue to ignore the obvious signs until we overstress and potentially damage ourselves.

In addition to getting a good night's rest, I suggest taking power naps, twenty minutes maximum, a few days a week in the early afternoon. These power naps energize most people, refresh your nerve system and help your body deal better with the effects of stress. This will help to give your body a needed energy boost.

Proper sleep increases healthy cellular function. While you sleep your blood is actually being cleansed and your body rebuilds, repairs and rejuvenates itself. Improve the quality of your sleep by purchasing the best mattress that your money can buy. There is nothing worst than a bad mattress. After sleeping on one, not only does you body feel robbed, but your spine is usually pretty messed up too which causes major problems to your overall health. Get a mattress that supports your weight and body size. I routinely recommend Select Comfort, and Tempur-Pedic mattresses or a firm regular mattress, which has a Tempur-Pedic-type foam top.

A proper pillow is essential as well for restful sleep. 80% of my patients sleep on an inadequate pillow usually one that is too soft and too low. Sleep preferably on your back or side with a pillow that is high enough to take up the space between your ear and the outside edge of your shoulder. I sleep on a Tempur-Pedic pillow myself and even travel with it. Also I recommend high quality feather pillows. Good pillows are more expensive, but play an important role in health and rarely need replacing.

Another thought is that you should sleep in a room that is totally dark. We are all big boys and girls now, and no longer need to sleep with the lights on. Actually a darkened environment sends a message to your body that you are ready to shut down and receive an uninterrupted replenishing. Lights send a message to your body that you need to be doing something since that is the general idea of having lights on in the first place. Rest gives you back your energy. Remember if you don't choose to get rest, your body will choose for you, hopefully not permanent rest.

Lose Weight

Having too much weight on your body, around your heart and around your waist will always cause you to feel tired. Even ten pounds of extra weight is a burden to carry around and steals energy. If you had to carry around a five pound bag of sugar or flour in each hand for a few hours you would quickly begin to see and feel my point. Many people are carrying around far more than ten extra pounds actually about two thirds of the adult population. We were not designed to carry those excess pounds.. Our body in fit shape, is the weight that God designed for us to carry, no more than that. Extra weight always saps your energy as you are causing your body to work harder in every area.

Some people who are overweight are so because they continue to make excuses about why they cannot lose weight. There are literally hundreds of different weight loss plans. I believe that the majority of them work if you follow the plan step by step. I believe in the simple yet proven weight loss strategy ELEM, which stands for eat less and exercise more. Find the weight plan that works best for you, be disciplined and work it. Portion control, making wiser food choices and getting more physical activity is the key to long term weight control and management.

Learn the Power of Saying "No"

Slow down your life by simplifying your life. Noted author Dr. Myles Munroe said, "God designed for your life to be simple." He believes that we need to simplify our life down to one thing, possibly two that we put most of our attention and energy into. When you try to do everything, not only will you be drained, you won't do well at anything. One of the things that you must realize is that most everything seems to matter in life. The question is what matters most? When the things that matter the most have to suffer for the things that matter least, then unnecessary energy, has been exerted, and in most cases is wasted.

Just learn how to say no. In my town and in my profession I am fairly well known. I have been offered opportunities that really appeared to be good propositions at first look, but then I had to look a bit harder. I ask myself this question, "Is what I'm being offered going to enhance or support what I am already actively doing?" If the answer is no, then my answer will be no. I cannot do everything and still expect to be an excellent chiropractor, husband, father and leader, which are my truest intentions. So then everything that I am offered has to fit within the framework of what I believe I am called to do in life.

It may be a good idea but is it God's idea? You will be offered many opportunities in life, some good and some not so good. I can assure you that if you accept them just to save someone from feeling bad or to try and see if it'll work, you will end up with even higher levels of stress, which will exacerbate your low energy crisis even further. If it does not fit within the context of your program, say no. There is only one of you. And you have to learn to preserve your most valuable asset, you.

A crowded mind is a difficult place to grow healthy thoughts.

A crowded mind is a difficult place to grow healthy thoughts. Simplify your life, decrease your schedule, and delegate out some of your work to others. Maybe you are one of those persons who believe that if you don't do it then it won't get done. Believe me when I tell you that is simply untrue. If you were dead, life will still go on, and whatever needed to get done would get done. Don't die trying to prove me wrong.

CHAPTER THREE

Losing Weight Naturally

———→•◦•←———

L et's talk candidly about the subject of losing weight. Obesity has unquestionably become a universal problem. However, in the United States of America it has become a problem that continues to escalate rapidly, perhaps far quicker than other nations. According to the National Center for Health Statistics 30 percent of the adults in America (60 million people) over 20 years of age, are obese. If that's not bad enough, 16 percent (more than nine million) of the children in between the ages of 6 – 19 are overweight. Personally, I believe that these figures are lower than what really is factual. However, between those two statistical figures, more than a quarter of the population in the United States is overweight.

The clothing industry has accommodated the growing trends in overweight fashion. Some of the most fashionable clothing lines come only in big sizes, helping to perpetuate and in some cases exploit the declining health condition of many obese people. The problem is so big that there are even fat resorts. These are vacation spots that are made to accommodate the very overweight. These resorts are a growing trend and include larger doorways, oversize chaise lounges poolside, bigger beds, armless chairs and the like. Don't go taking this the wrong way. I am not trying to put a guilt trip on you, or make you believe that everybody in the world has to be picture perfect or perfectly thin for that matter. Slender and perfectly fit is not my ultimate goal here. Most of the weight loss advertisements and television infomercials show a person who is in incredibly fit shape with a nearly unachievable body with ripped abs, muscular body, buns of steel, bikini or Speedo clad who walks off into the sunset holding hands with the new found man or woman of their dreams. That sells weight loss products but that's not my goal for you.

I am a slim guy, but I don't have an abdominal section like Arnold Schwarznegger, and 36-inch biceps to match, neither do I have any desire to go there. One thing that I can truthfully say though, is that I am healthy, very healthy at that. I am healthy and fit because I have chosen to be. And if you listen to what I am going to teach you, you too can experience amazing wellness. Remember that looks can be very deceiving. Not everybody that has a sculpted body is necessarily in good health.

Many athletes, models, and bodybuilders have major health problems, simply because they over do it in one area, typically the area of working out or in dieting for the wrong reasons, while they tend to neglect many of the other areas that are equally as important. It's not necessarily my concern how great you look in your two-piece bathing suit, or your Tommy Bahama

...why lose weight? ...so you won't die early!

shorts though that may be a nice side benefit of following my advice. How you look is totally your personal preference. How it will make you feel about yourself and how it will make you feel physically though, is my concern, my burden, and it will continue to be that way until you start living the life that you deserve.

Well if losing weight is not primarily about the look then, why lose weight? Answer, so you won't die early! As quiet as it is kept, being overweight is no laughing matter. If left unchecked it can and will spawn a multitude of health problems and various diseases in the body that will eventually lead to your early death. Your medical doctor may not have the courage or the understanding to be that blunt with you until it's too late. What I mean by too late is waiting to be that honest before serious damage and sometimes irreparable damage is done. They too often will tell you to lose weight, when your body is so damaged and destroyed by arthritis, pain and fatigue that there is very little that you can do except take their drugs.

After a couple of strokes or major heart attacks, you won't feel much like surfing, snowboarding, or even walking the dog for that matter. That's what I mean by too late. Okay, I may appear to be a bit sarcastic, but this is your life that I am talking about. And I care. So if you can just get over my straightforward approach, you'll really get something out of all this—LIFE. And that is what I intend to give you. So you need to lose weight, for one reason. Come on, say it aloud, TO LIVE. Obesity kills! Being significantly overweight leads and is a precursor (interesting word) to many fatal diseases such as:

- Colon Cancer
- Stroke
- Liver and Gallbladder Disease
- Heart Disease (which inevitably leads to heart attacks)
- Breathing Problems
- Osteoporosis
- Sky High Cholesterol
- Diabetes

And that's only an abridged list. I hope that I am motivating you to at least consider some of the most valid reasons for getting and/or keeping your weight under control. But if you need to lose weight don't go out and start making unwise decisions with your health. In America typically when people need to lose weight, they want to do it as fast and easy as possible with the least pain possible, the fast food approach to weight loss. The fast food approach simply says, I want to lose weight, I want it now and I am in a hurry. After all your sister's wedding or your family vacation to the beach is only a month away, right?

Give me a number two; no make that a number three weight loss program. I'll take it to go, and I expect incredible results, overnight. I advise you to slow down, stop and think first. Some diets may give you the slim and trim results quickly, but they'll also give you something else, more weight and put you in worse health than before. So you have to be very careful about what you put into your body. Every diet is not a diet made in heaven although some may get you there a whole lot sooner than you expected.

Diet Plans Can Kill

There are some diet approaches that can kill you, no matter which way you look at it, and should be avoided at all cost. I won't attempt to name them all as they are countless but I will highlight a few for your safety. Hastiness inevitably leads to making wrong decisions, and causing your body more damage than it had to begin with. So the first thing you should know, is that the majority of the time you do have good choices. I realize that some of you are feeling in a state of emergency, but truthfully, you were in that same state before I told you how bad off you were. Take time to research the healthiest all-natural, drug and surgery free alternative for you.

With that said, here are a few diets to avoid. *Fasting* diets should be avoided at all cost. I am not saying that you should not fast. Fasting is a spiritual and naturopathic discipline that has had proven results in the areas of greater spiritual awareness and inner cleansing. So first off, fasting should be done, for one of those two reasons, either for spiritual benefits, or to detoxify your toxic system. Aside from those two reasons fasting, typically for weight loss purposes, especially for long periods of continuous days or weeks can be extremely dangerous.

What happens exactly when you fast? First, you begin to lose weight quickly which is why many people desperately choose this method. That's the obvious. The unobvious is when you fast your body begins to feed off of itself since there is no food going into it. When that happens you begin to lose muscle instead of the fat tissue that you so desperately want and need to lose. On the outside everything looks pretty favorable. Your friends and family members will tell you how great you are beginning to look. However, what you cannot feel and they cannot see is the major damage happening on your inside.

Your muscle is the metabolic workhorse in your body that helps to burn the fat off. So when you lose muscle you slow down your internal metabolism permanently. No one that knows anything about slow metabolism wants anything to do with it. It's like firing for no legitimate reason, your internal head coach of fat burning. Then when you start eating again, which at some point you obviously will, you'll find that you eventually gain back more weight than you had before. However this time around, you are powerless to overcome it because of your declining metabolism. If that

All drugs should be avoided whenever possible and especially for weight loss.
∼

is over your head just know it is counterproductive. Don't do it. It is an unhealthy approach.

Another method that has proven to be a fatal weight loss method is *diet drugs*. No matter how you look at it, drugs are drugs. Diet drugs like all other drugs don't get to the root of the problem but only attempt to chemically alter the body. All drugs should be avoided whenever possible and especially for weight loss. Herbs sold on infomercials are no better. The way diet drugs and diet herbs work is quite similar to how David Blaine, the great Houdini, and David Copperfield work, they play tricks on your mind. It's called an illusion. They chemically make your brain believe you're your full and satisfied by altering brain chemistry,and there is always a downside.

There is a recently popular diet developed by a now famous and deceased medical doctor that tells people that it is OK to eat all the meat and animal fat they want like steak, pork, bacon, sausage, etc. This eat all the red meat and fat diet is ludicrous. Come on, I don't care how many letters you have or don't have behind your name; you know that doesn't make any sense at all. You don't need a college degree to figure that out. Ingesting high levels of red meat and animal fat will still have the same unhealthy side effects as it always has had. Fat clogs your veins and arteries making it difficult for blood to flow freely and causes colon cancer. Although this diet has been successful in causing many people to lose weight, it should too be known that one deviation from the diet as prescribed can cause your body to go into a sudden downward spiraling affect. It's not worth it.

Fat-free and extremely low calorie diets can be just as harmful as the "eat more meat and fat" diets. Remember everything should be done in moderation. Unless you are extremely overweight and under the supervision of a qualified health practitioner you should not pursue a low calorie diet, and never a fat-free diet as there are many good fats containing very important essential fatty acids that your body needs and cannot get any other way.

Avoid also the *one extreme to the other extreme* diets, these diets suggest extremely high protein or carbohydrate intake or extremely low protein or carbohydrate intake.

Both extremes can be harmful, as you will lose the building blocks needed for long-term good health in the process.

Let's just face it. Diets don't work. They are dangerous and a Band-Aid to the real problem. The best method to lose weight once and for all is lifestyle change backed by the desire for a healthy, long life.. It's not as important to abruptly change, as it is to know and understand the reason for your change. That way you'll get out of the rut and stay out, for good. If you made enough change to lose even one pound a week in fifty two weeks you will have lost fifty two pounds.

How Did It All Happen?

To lose weight you must first understand how you got into that situation in the first place. How and why did you gain the weight? It did not just appear there by osmosis. There are a number of possible reasons that you may be predisposed to being overweight. Let's list just a few.

- You have a genetic predisposition to weight gain
- Your family is obese.
- You recently had a baby.
- You are going through menopause.
- You have a thyroid problem.
- You were injured in an accident and cannot exercise as you used to.

- You have a serious health issue or became sick.

- You have a sedentary lifestyle.

- You have low self esteem.

These are all very legitimate reasons however don't let them also become excuses. If you are affected by any of these you must be even more diligent in your efforts and more firm in your resolve to take control of your life before things get even one step worse. The best things in life always require discipline, preparation, and patience. If the reason why you are overweight is connected to one or more of these areas honesty with yourself is and will always be the best policy.

I believe that the reasons listed below, represent a closer to reality picture of why you may not be where you'd like to be weight-wise. Believe me when I tell you that the sooner you accept the truth, and the sooner you are honest with yourself the sooner you'll be on the road to true wellness and a longer life.

The Real Deal—I have weight management issues because . . .

- ❏ I eat the wrong foods.

- ❏ I don't exercise or don't take exercising seriously.

- ❏ I am under too much stress.

- ❏ I rarely or never get enough sleep.

❑ I have a poor metabolism or slow metabolism.

❑ I lack self discipline.

❑ I don't care enough about myself.

❑ I am addicted to sugar.

❑ I am addicted to caffeine.

❑ I don't take the time to prepare healthy meals.

If you checked one or more of these possible reasons then I am sure that you are beginning the process of being honest with yourself. Also, I am convinced that you really are serious about getting to the body you deserve. I'll offer you some practical starters before we close this chapter out, but for now let me offer you some hope. Your body innately knows how to keep your weight at its proper amount and in proportional alignment with the rest of your body, when it is working properly.

So let's chat a minute about two very important pieces to your body operating properly. The first is that your nervous system controls and coordinates all the function in your body. For your nerve system to work optimally, your spine needs to be well-aligned, strong, and healthy. That is what I have spent the majority of my career teaching people. You don't typically hear about healthy spines with regard to proper weight management. I have had any number of patients come to me with allergy, sinus, back, neck or various other issues and within two or three months they begin losing significant weight as their body begins to work out it's own inner balance issues all by itself. I cannot understate the importance of a healthy spine in all aspects of your health because it is your most important health ally. An unhealthy spine is an inciter of many body problems. Let's talk about the other major issue that most authors of diet books are clueless about.

Maintaining A Healthy Liver

There are literally hundreds of thousands of seminars, workshops and interactive discussions on various topics about weight loss. From muscle toning, to eating the right natural foods, to drinking plenty of distilled water, to breathing deeply in several times daily to filling those lungs with clean fresh air, it seems like we've heard it all. Yet strangely enough, we don't hear anything about the liver. It is one of your most important organs.

So what's so important about the liver? First, your liver is the largest organ in your body weighing in at 3 lbs. on average. It sits just above the right corner of your abdomen. It performs some very complex functions necessary for life and healing. Look at your liver as a filter for your bloodstream and as an internal chemical processing plant. Unlike your arms and legs, eyes, or ears, you cannot live without your liver.

What does your liver have to do with weight management and weight loss? There are far more things that the liver does, enough to write an entire book on. But for now, I would just like to concentrate on its nutritional contribution to your body. Literally everything that you eat, junk food, candy, medications, vitamins or even your favorite Italian, Thai, or Mexican dish, gets absorbed through the walls of your stomach and intestines and is then processed in some way or detoxified by your liver. That is why proper nutrition matters, since what you put in you will inevitably come out of you or become some part of your anatomy.

Here are some of things that the liver does: ***Your Liver...***

- Has more than 400 different jobs

- Regulates blood sugar

- Controls hormone balance

- Converts your food into energy

- Filters toxic substances from the blood and converts them into waste matter

- Produces immune system factors

- Makes proteins and enzymes necessary for production and transport of hormones in the bloodstream

- Makes cholesterol, an essential substance for healthy nerve function

- Produces chemicals essential for growth and anatomical development

In addition to that is also:

- Produces 1 quart of yellow-green fluid called bile per day
- Bile is stored by the gall bladder and is released into the intestine
- Bile emulsifies, digests fat

Realizing just how important your liver is, you really don't want to put additional stress on it. It already has a hard enough job. So when you put added stress on your liver, it compromises its ability to perform normally. Liver neglect usually costs your life. So below I've listed some things that always brings unnecessary stress into your liver. Avoid them!

These Things Stress Your Liver —

- Caffeine
- Sugar—which, causes inflammation, high insulin
- Trans Fats—overworks it causing a rise in both good and bad cholesterol levels
- Prescription Medicine—many of which can severely harm it
- Inadequate fiber in your diet—fiber helps to remove toxins, increase bowel movement speed, cleans the bowel for better absorption, absorbs water in bowel, and lowers cholesterol

Exercise

Weight loss and exercise go hand in hand. Don't miss this important step. Exercise has so many obvious benefits such as improving your sleep, burning unwanted and unneeded calories, raising your metabolism, improving your digestion, and increasing the speed of fecal matter through the intestines. It helps flush your lymphatic system which helps you to eliminate wastes and toxins quickly and efficiently. Exercise also oxygenates your tissues, wards off stress, and increases your endorphin production. The benefits are unlimited. So start doing some physical activity that you enjoy or something as simple as bouncing on a mini-trampoline 5 minutes a day. Or maybe you can do brisk walking with brisk arm movements 15 to twenty minutes daily. Even a little exercise is better than no exercise.

Supplementation

In a forthcoming chapter, Chapter Eight, *Vitamin Supplements—Where Do I Begin*, I will deal in more detail with what vitamins that are truly essential for everyday living from vitamins which you should take every now and then. But for now, I have listed a recommendation of supplements that will immediately begin working on your liver.

Supplements

a. Flax Seed Oil 1-2tbs/day

   1) helps liver function

2) provides Omega 3 essential fatty acids

3) helps hormone production and regulation

4) improves heart health, circulation

5) reduces pain and inflammation

b. GLA Evening Primrose, Borage, Black Current Seed Oil (alternate with Flax Seed Oil)

1) provides Omega 3 and 6 Essential Fatty Acids

c. Multi-Vitamin and Mineral Supplement (natural not synthetic)

d. Livaplex 2/day (a supplement from the Standard Process company)

1) Helps clean your liver

2) Supports healthy bile production

e. Symplex M or F (M for males or F for females also from Standard Process)

1) For healthy hormone production

Detoxification

In order for you to get your liver working optimally you are going to have to detoxify your liver. If you drive a car, about every 3000 to 5000 miles you have to get an oil change, lube and filter as they say. If you choose to wait until the 100,000 mile point to get an oil change, your engine (if it is still operable) may end up needing a total overhaul, perhaps it may need to be rebuilt in order to work. Most people's livers are in a similar condition to a car engine that's not been well taken care of. The good news is that the body is far more forgiving than your car. If you begin now making the necessary changes needed, within a small amount of time you will begin to experience changes that are not only visible but can be felt deep within. The following suggestions will help you to eliminate cellulite, get your liver pure and help remove toxins out of your body. Here is your liver cleanse formula.

To Help Detoxify and Cleanse Your Liver and Lymphatic System

a. Hot water plus the juice from ½ lemon twice per day

b. Cranberry Water Flush

   1) 4oz. unsweetened cranberry juice + 28oz. pure water = 32oz. Drink 64oz. total per day

   2) Flushes lymphatic system

   3) Reduces cellulite

c. Fiber Booster (if you can't eat enough steamed and raw vegetables)

   1) 8oz. cranberry water described above plus 1 tsp. psyllium husks or 1 Tbsp. of ground flax seeds

d. ½ apple a day-pectin in the apple helps to keep bile thin

Getting Started—Making Weight Loss Natural and Simple

Let's de-mystify this whole weight loss thing and give some practical what-to-do tips that will serve you well for the rest of your life. Weight management does not have to be complicated nor complex. It's pretty much as easy as you accept it to be. Here is a list, of things I suggest in my wellness seminars and regularly recommend to my patients. These steps have yielded remarkable results when followed diligently. Start by getting on the scale and deciding that you will never weigh more than you weigh today. This one tip is how I began to control my weight.

In addition...

Dr. Madeira's Natural Weight Loss Plan

- Stop Drinking Soda forever-diet and regular

- Eat Smaller Portions more often-minimizes insulin release which causes fat storage on your body

- Drink More Pure Water – start by drinking more per day than whatever you are drinking now-not from the tap

- Start Exercising a little everyday-start small if you have to

- Stop Eating Trans Fats especially margarines, butter substitutes, commercial peanut butters and french fries most all of which are full of trans fat (aka partially hydrogenated oils)

- Eliminate Processed Foods—don't eat anything you can't pronounce

- Eliminate the White Family—white sugar, white flour, white rice, white bread

- Increase Your Fiber Intake by eating many more steamed and raw vegetables

- Eat 8 oz. of Lean Protein per day plus eat two eggs per day

- Wean Off of Coffee—get down to 1 cup per day-none if possible.

- Portion Your Food in the kitchen but eat in the dining room—decide beforehand how much you want to eat—don't have seconds

- Get On the Scale every morning—knowing where you are at the start of each day helps keep you honest with yourself

CHAPTER FOUR

How To Boost Your Immune System

Your immune system is one of the most complex and vitally important aspects of the human body. It is so complex that even the most skilled medical practitioners, Chiropractors, and research experts have not yet figured out every element of its inner workings. It is safe to postulate that no one person will ever have a comprehensive understanding of this vast topic, since the body is such an intricate masterpiece. It is like an onion, which reveals deeper and deeper layers of complexity as it is peeled. For every question that some expensive research study answers five new unanswered questions are revealed which we never even thought to ask.

At best many health care professionals can explain how the body systems work but in the event that some part of it fails they resort to the knowledge they were taught in medical school, which instinctively tells them to medicate or perform surgery much like a hammer that sees everything as a nail. While that method has become socially acceptable medicating people to treat ailments instead of offering natural healing alternatives is killing people. Most health professionals have at least a basic understanding of how the immune system works, but few actually know how to fix it when it breaks down. Fewer still know how to maximize its natural function. That is what this chapter is all about.

> *Our bodies are amazing healing machines when they are working properly.*

Our bodies are amazing healing machines when they are working properly. They are built to resist disease and to fix and repair most of the common everyday things that can go wrong with a human body without any outside help. Once we understand how healing happens in the body and what controls it we can then work with the design to help optimize its function. When you finish reading this portion of the book you will know exactly what to do to maximize your own immune resistance. You will have a better understanding of how to boost and strengthen the human immune system than most family physicians, guaranteed.

As an example let's say that you drive a Lexus automobile. Lexus has established a long-standing reputation for building quality automobiles that outlast its competition. If you've ever owned a Lexus you know that your car rarely goes to the shop other than for routine maintenance such as oil changes, tire rotations and changing the filters. Very rarely will you see a late model Lexus go to the shop for reasons such as engine, transmission or mechanical failure.

This is not a paid advertisement for Lexus. It is only a clear illustration to help explain my point. Lexus, unlike many of its competitors was not a car designed to be in the shop. You're probably asking, "What types of cars are actually made to go to the shop?" The answer to that question is simply too many. In fact, there are a number of brands of automobiles that are made to be disposable with the clear intention of getting you to buy replacement vehicles repeatedly and/or pay for frequent repairs. Let's face it we have the technology and know how to build things to last much longer than they typically do.

Companies that choose to build inferior cars, rarely offer worthwhile warranties on their products knowing that they'll end up paying out so much in repair costs that it will actually have an adverse affect on their profit margin. So they build cars for cheap and sell it to you for cheap. When it breaks down, and it will, you won't bicker too much about it, because you paid so little up front. You may actually end up paying more in time, money, and lost opportunities than the Lexus owner, who chose to pay the larger cost up front but did not have to deal with the high expense and inconvenience of unending auto repairs.

Many people actually spend more energy maintaining their car than their own body.

~

If the car manufacturers built their cars with quality to begin with then you would not really have to worry about major breakdowns, only regularly scheduled tune-ups and maintenance. The human body can be viewed in the same way as the Lexus. It was built by the hands of a master craftsman and designed to last. Of course it will stay in that same shape if you use high octane fuel in the form of the highest quality nutrients and mineral rich food available, and have regularly scheduled maintenance visits with your chiropractor. Many people actually spend more energy maintaining their car than their own body. Imagine that!

I'm not saying that negative things cannot happen to your health unexpectedly. However, taking great care of yourself will drastically reduce the odds of that happening. Your body was designed to actually heal itself. When things are working together in harmony that is exactly what happens. So if you properly maintain your body your immune system will function optimally. If you do not, then you will inevitably experience a system failure sooner or later. It is not a matter of if but when.

When that happens, you will instinctively seek out professionals, to help to get you up and going again. So when your immune system is weakened what does is need? It needs the things that would have caused it not to fail in the first place. Does that make sense to you? In other words, if taking drugs every day would strengthen your immune system, then that would mean most people that are sick suffer from a drug intake deficiency. Okay, I'm being a bit sarcastic. I'm only trying to get you to actually see how ridiculous many people behave and how irrationally they think when it comes to their health. Your body was not made with a drug deficiency.

If your car runs out of gas on the side of the road, you wouldn't phone the American Automobile Association (AAA) and ask them to send a flat bed tow truck with a table filled with gourmet food because your car is really hungry. No you would ask them to send a truck with about 5 gallons of gas. When your car stalls in order to get it going again you have to give it what it needs to continue on. No one's body functions from the use of drugs. Perhaps some people use drugs because their body is so depleted or damaged that they have no other choice, but even then the drugs may only band-aid the problem and sustain them until they die, but that's all. The drugs don't' heal or fix them. Even in those situations when a drug(s) is necessary to keep someone alive those drugs have other effects, harmful effects. So don't rely on pretty pills or magical surgeries to bail you out in the end. That is a smooth and slippery slope that too often ends in a huge gamble. Commit now to take better care of yourself.

Your Immune System

I want you to have a basic understanding of what your immune system is. It's very important for you to know what it is and how it works. Most people know what the weather forecast will be for the day. Guys typically know what last night's game scores were for the sport team they most love. Investors carefully scrutinize what's going on in the stock market from day to day. Many women, (and men too) know about the sales at Neiman Marcus and Macy's, yet few people know much about why their immune system is so important.

Your body, your organs, and even your skin are constantly exposed to stress, elements in the atmosphere such as pollutants and toxins, extreme temperature changes and invasion by foreign organisms each of which can cause major impact and damage. Your body has several very fascinating built in ways of guarding itself from potentially harmful substances. For example, dogs can easily get fleas running around outside and rolling in the grass, so caring pet owners can spray their dogs with flea spray as a preventative measure. The flea spray acts as a repellant and a protective agent against the fleas.

The chemicals in the spray repel the fleas and ticks from latching onto the dog. In the same way, your immune system is a very strategic network of thousands of cells that immediately recognize foreign and unwelcome substances in the body and launches a literal war against them, ultimately killing them. This literal police force of cells is armed and dangerous and kills foreign cells, parasites, even cancer cells before they get the chance to organize and reproduce. This process like the police in your town are constantly watching for the bad guys and handling the problem before they ever get started.

Suppose your immune system just ignores the intruder or allows them to just hang out for a while, then what? What if your immune system and therefore your immune resistance is weakened, tired, or extremely suppressed? When that happens it may not be strong enough to protect you, let alone fight against potential predators, sickness and disease trying to enter in. If your body remains suppressed you open the door to disease, lots of suffering and even potentially a premature death.

Here is a list of some of the diseases that a healthy immune system helps to fight against:

- Colds, Viruses, Sore Throats and Flu

- Infections of the Eyes, Ears, Nose and Throat

- Infections of the Organs such as Heart, Lungs, Bladder, Kidneys

- Childhood Diseases like Whooping Cough, Measles, Chicken Pox

- Sexually Transmitted Diseases

- All Types of Cancer

- Allergies, Asthma, Sinusitis and Bronchitis

- Auto-Immune Disorders Like Lupus and Rheumatoid Arthritis

- Chronic Fatigue Syndrome and Fibromyalgia

- Aids, SARS, The Bird Flu and Similar Plague-like Diseases

Doing It The Natural Way

The best way to build your immune system is to do it naturally. When you build your immune system in that way, you never have to worry about adverse reactions or negative side effects. Building natural immunity is always better. It is time to teach you six specific things you can do to improve your body's ability to stay well and fight off infection and disease.

Adjust it! Getting your spine adjusted (re-aligned) has a profound effect on your immune resistance and is absolutely the number one best thing you can do on a regular basis to boost your own immunity. Your immune system is a direct extension of your nerve system. The nerve system is what carries the signals or messages from your brain to the rest of your body. Getting your spine checked and kept in strong, healthy alignment is by far the most often overlooked and under-investigated aspect of strong immunity. It is uncertain exactly how but is absolutely clear that people with healthy strong spines have massively healthier immune systems. People who go the Chiropractor for regular wellness re-alignments or spinal adjustments as they are called are among the healthiest people on the planet. They enjoy amazing levels of heath and extremely lower incidences of cancer, heart disease, strokes and other catastrophic diseases.

It is unclear exactly how but it is extremely clear that regular Chiropractic care prevents cancer, heart disease and strokes.

Each nerve signal sent from the brain gives the body direction and tells it what it needs to do. For example it tells the bone marrow to produce more of a particular kind of white blood cell to fight off a certain kind of foreign invader. It tells the white blood cells where to go to begin the miraculous work of healing you in specific areas of need. It helps direct it there by dilating blood vessels to those areas that need more infection fighters, oxygen and nutrients on the scene in the same way a police dispatcher immediately sends the police to the scene of a crime or accident scene.

Feed it! Feeding your body organic, antioxidant-rich, nutrient strong foods especially fresh green leafy vegetables, fruit, and foods high in vitamins A, B, C, D and E, help to strengthen your immune system. They act as specialists, dealing with specific areas in your body. For example:

- Vitamin A—counteracts weakened eyesight, and aids in the treatment of various eye disorders, helps the immune system to function properly, shortens the length of diseases, removes age spots, promotes growth of strong bones, healthy skin, teeth, and gums

- Vitamin B—B complex vitamins improve your mental system, keep muscles, heart, and nervous system functioning properly, improves cellular function

- Vitamin C—helps to lower your cholesterol, heals wounds and burns, helps to prevent viral and bacterial infections, protects against cancer-causing agents, acts as a natural laxative, strengthens cellular function, fights against allergy producers, supports the immune system, natural anti-oxidant, and strengthens blood vessels

- Vitamin D—when taken with vitamins A and C it helps in preventing colds and helps the body absorb calcium for strong bones

- Vitamin E—retards cellular aging helping to keep you looking younger, aids in keeping skin healthy, gives you greater endurance by supplying oxygen to the body, alleviates fatigue, dissolves blood clots, accelerates the healing of burns, lowers blood pressure, and helps decrease the risk of heart disease

Depending on the person, some of these vitamins may be needed in higher milligram dosages. Everybody's needs are quite different, so it is important for you to get to know your body, how it works, and what it needs at this particular time in your life. Even as you grow older there are certain things that you need more of later in life than you did when you were younger. For example, seniors typically require less sleep than people in their young and mid adult years since they are not as active, and require less recharging time.

In addition to the list of primary vitamins there are a few things that are not as widely known, that can also be very helpful in strengthening your overall immune system.

- Selenium—helps to keep your tissues youthful and elastic, it may neutralize certain cancer causing agents and provide protection against some cancers, can be found in seafood, kidney, liver, bran, tuna fish, onions, broccoli, and wheat germ

- Pine bark extract—a powerful antioxidant and known arthritis aid

- Grape seed extract—helps to improve cardiovascular health, promotes brain, skin, and eye health, improves mental alertness, prevents senility, and arthritis helper

- Grapefruit seed extract—antioxidant with natural anti-viral, anti-bacterial and anti-fungal properties

Breastfeed it! Babies that are breastfed tend to be far healthier than babies that are fed synthetic formulas out of a can or box. The vitamins and nutrients in natural breast milk contain powerful antibodies that get passed from mother to child. These antibodies and other immunity factors are natural immune building blocks, which provide an important foundation for strong lifelong immunity. Liquid and powder formulas are a poor simulation of the real thing. They attempt to provide the same benefits of natural breast milk but fall far short of that goal. Breast-feeding stimulates brain growth and all the psychological and emotional benefits a plastic nipple will never afford. Breast milk is so nutrient and vitamin rich, that Olympians actually use it to train for their races and sports events, paying very high prices for it.

My wife and I adopted both of our children. Because breast milk was not available we raised them on pure goat's milk from a local goat farm. Every week we would make a trip to the Red Gate Goat Farm for another supply. Raw goat milk is the next best thing to human mother's milk. Both our children have grown into wonderful healthy young adults with strong bones and healthy teeth and immune systems. Another decision we made after intense information gathering was to not vaccinate our children.

Don't vaccinate it! More and more, people are becoming aware of the real truth concerning vaccinations. In my opinion vaccines are a gross assault on an immature

More and more, people are becoming aware of the real truth concerning vaccinations.

immune system. I realize that my opinion is somewhat controversial in the eyes of Big Brother Medicine but I am just not convinced that injecting monkey pus and other live, attenuated or dead infectious animal products is a healthy thing to do. In America, generally all children are required to get vaccinations. In fact, most public schools and colleges threaten to not allow your child to come to school until they've had all of their shots. They even threaten that it is illegal to be admitted to school without them, though that is not the case in most states. Be aware that most states do allow exemptions for parents with strong convictions against vaccinations. While mass inoculations are commonly accepted and routine, they are drastically harming the overall health of our children. Vaccinations actually work against the body's natural ability to heal itself. They break down the immune system rather than build it up.

By the time that a child turns 4 years old, they have had more than 77 toxic substances injected into their immature immune system, starting the second day of their life. That's craziness and insanity. The big question is do vaccinations work?

There is some proof that vaccines stimulate antibodies to form against specific invaders. They too often are only temporary and oft times harmful. There is tremendous argument and controversy about the drastic rise in Autism and its direct link to vaccine use. I believe there is a direct link. Most naturally-minded health care professionals agree with my opinion. It is hard to deny. Yet the drug companies and the medical profession grossly deny any connection. Of course they do.

My Amish patients have taught me a lot about the effectiveness of vaccines and the practice of mass inoculation. Amish babies are born at home by midwives and they don't vaccinate their children. I can count on one hand the number of my Amish patients that have asthma, allergies or sinus problems. In those few rare instances the person was vaccinated as a child when they were in the hospital for one reason or another.

Sudden Infant Death Syndrome or Crib Death as it is sometimes called has been directly implicated in mass inoculation efforts yet SIDS and Autism are virtually non-existent among the Amish. They don't even know what Autism is. It does not take a rocket scientist to see the obvious here. They don't trust medical doctors as a general rule and avoid vaccines, drugs and hospitals whenever possible.

On the other hand among my regular non-Amish patients, allergies and sinus problems are the rule rather than the exception. "Hello McFly" is anyone listening? Asthma cases are dramatically on the increase yet no one wants to admit the connection. 100,000 people die yearly from asthma and its complications and it is rising. Is anybody home in the CDC (Centers for Disease Control)? I have cared for thousands over twenty five years. These statements are no exaggeration.

Vaccinations are not the only way to achieve the same goal. Our bodies were given the mechanisms to create natural and permanent immunity if they are only allowed to be exposed naturally. Before drugging up yourself and your children, begin to check out resources that will help you gain a clearer understanding about what options you have. Strangely, vaccines end up causing damage to the immune system by weakening it. To find out more about vaccines check out the National Vaccine Information Center at www.909shot.com. This is an excellent place to begin your due diligence on vaccines and their potential dangers especially for new moms and dads or new moms and dads to be. Another great resource is Pediatrician Dr. Stephanie Cave's book *What Your Doctor May Not Tell You About Children's Vaccinations*. In it she presents a balanced middle of the road approach to vaccinating your children. I highly recommend it.

> *...many people fail to realize is that, not some, but every drug has negative side affects to it.*

Don't medicate it! Stop taking drugs for every problem and ailment that happens in your body, especially antibiotics which prevent your body from building permanent immunity. Drugs can become very addictive. And what many people fail to realize is that, not some, but every drug has negative side affects to it. Some drugs have been even known to create super infections. Prescribing antibiotics for every little cold and sore throat that comes along has actually caused bacteria to adapt and become immune. This ability to adapt is at the core of every living organism and is so powerful that some bacteria have actually begun thriving on antibiotic medication as if it is food. This has created a dilemma known as superinfections, bacterial infections that are totally resistant to antibiotics.

If you listen carefully to any drug advertisement on television, you will hear at the end of the commercial the long list of possible side affects that the drug causes. Why take a drug to help lower your blood pressure, or lower your cholesterol yet simultaneously the same drug is causing you to have renal failure, heart palpitations, and sexual dysfunction. It may also cause stomach pain, ulcers and induce vomiting. The trade off is an unfair one. Drugs do not support the immune system. So its better to avoid them at all cost.

Exercise it! Regular exercise also builds the immune system through increased tissue strength, improved circulation of blood and lymph systems and improved oxygenation of nearly all body tissues. This is just one more reason to get those running shoes, golf clubs and tennis racquets out of the garage.

Lets recap the six things you can do to naturally help strengthen your own immune system:

- Adjust it!
- Feed it!
- Breastfeed it!
- Don't vaccinate it!
- Don't medicate it!
- Exercise it!

The Germ Theory

The germ theory is a theory from ancient times that states that anyone who comes in contact with a germ of any kind will automatically get sick from coming in contact with it. The whole practice of medicine is based on it and it is a false theory. Germs do not cause disease any more than flies cause garbage. Healthy people have healthy tissues. Only unhealthy people get sick. The very healthy may develop something simple like the common cold, a sore throat or at worst the stomach flu but rarely anything worse. People who are truly strong and healthy on the inside do not drop over dead from heart attacks or get cancer. Only those whose inner health has slowly deteriorated and whose resistance has become compromised get sick with serious illness. There is always a reason why someone becomes sick or gets diagnosed with a disease, always.

If the germ theory was true no one who works in a hospital would be alive to talk about it.

If the germ theory was true no one who works in a hospital would be alive to talk about it. All doctors, dentists and nurses would be dead. Health care workers are around germs and sick people all the time. Yet just the opposite occurs. They buildup resistance and rarely get sick.

As a child I remember going to the medical doctor when I was little and wanting to be a doctor because he was never sick. I thought there was something special about him. In fact there was, his immune system was exhibiting one of the many wonders of the human body. When your immune resistance is strong your body can deal with just about any bad bacteria, virus or parasite.

A new hypothesis now in vogue and getting much attention from the scientific community is called the Hygiene Hypothesis. It basically recognizes that sterile environments, antibacterial soaps, mass vaccine programs, etc. keep the immune system from getting any exercise. It would appear that the immune system needs to get exercise just like the rest of the body and when it doesn't it cannot build the strength and vitality required of it. People who live in less than sterile environments like farms and others who are allowed to play with other children who have or have been exposed to chicken pox and other childhood disorders actually have stronger immune systems and become sick less often. I see this with my Amish population of patients whose bodies are pure, free of vaccines, medicines, city air, and are around plenty of dirt and manure. Many have never been to a medical doctor and rely mostly on Chiropractors, home remedies and vitamin supplements for their health care.

Beware of These Things

Here is a listing of things that I call immune crashers. These things are guaranteed to adversely affect your immunes system.

- Unhealthy or improperly maintained spinal alignment

- Sugar

- Lack of regular sleep

- Heavy toxins such as mercury, fluoride, formaldehyde from vaccines and flu shots

- Heavy metals and toxins from air, water and food impurities

- Poor nutrition

- Toxic Relationships

Toxic relationships

This section on toxic relationships could be a book all by itself. It could also be a stage play or a full movie. This is the drama section of your life and how it relates to your overall health. You may wonder, what do toxic relationships have to do with your immune system? I believe that it has very much to do with your immune system. First, toxic relationships are simply draining. They pull on your emotions in the most negative way.

People involved in these relationships often lose unusual amounts of weight since they do not eat properly. They also, incur major amounts of stress and tension, which directly affect your nervous system. Also, these relationships can cause major sickness to develop within you. It is very necessary to re-evaluate your friendships from time to time. Ask yourself the question; am I receiving increase from being in a relationship with this person or decrease? The answer to that question can determine the outlook of your overall health.

Smoking

One of my common phrases that I've been known to say is, people are not stupid. People know right from wrong, but often choose to do what they should not. In terms of smoking, people have known for hundreds of years that smoking is hazardous to your health, yet they still light up. In 1604, King James I of England actually issued a censure against the use of tobacco. In more recent years a rising concern about the possibility of cigarettes causing health problems arose after World War II. Medical researchers then, began to compile all sorts of documentation to prove that smoking cigars and pipes can be directly linked to mouth and throat cancer and that smoking cigarettes can be linked to lung cancer.

Smoking also increases the risk of heart disease. It has been proven that smoking is an addictive drug. Although millions of people regularly smoke despite the warnings that are clearly written on each pack of cigarettes, smoking continues to compromise the strength of your immune system. In no short terms, smoking literally steals oxygen from you and exchanges it for noxious, addictive chemicals.

That's why you hear people choking and coughing heavily that are smokers. The reason they do so is because smoking takes your breath away. It takes your air from you. And since your immune system is totally dependent on fresh air and oxygen in order to function optimally, it is an unwise thing to ever consider smoking. And if you are already a smoker make a commitment to yourself to quit or begin to cut your cigarette consumption in half every month until you are completely free of it.

...make a commitment to yourself to quit or begin to cut your cigarette consumption in half every month...

Alcohol in Moderation

There are many viewpoints on alcohol consumption. The worst view on the subject has to do with the negative affects of alcoholism. While alcoholism is a universal problem, it definitely is greater in certain regions of the world than others. For example in Europe people drink alcohol with most meals. It is a part of their custom especially in countries like France, Spain, Italy and Portugal. If not taken to extremes it does not seem to cause obesity or other abundantly harmful effects.

For the most part the health of many people in these regions is relatively healthy employing this type of cultural diet. However in America, many people become excessive with alcohol consumption using it more as a drug to deal with stress, loneliness or heartache. This actually can lead to brain, liver and blood vessel damage and have other detrimental effects not excluding obesity. Overindulgence with regards to alcohol can also have very negative affects on your immune system. Use common sense, and learn to exercise control in this area and in any other area that may be potentially harmful to your health.

CHAPTER FIVE

Increasing Your Body's Ability To Heal Itself

In this chapter I want to deal with some major yet often overlooked aspects of healing and healthy living. There are many healing techniques that involve external involvement such as taking vitamins, exercise, and eating the right foods. All of those things are quite valuable, as we've already discussed so far in this book. However, just as important are the things that happen within, the intangible internals. There are some people that eat the right foods, and exercise daily yet find themselves dealing with major complications in their health.

As a rule they cannot figure out why they still get sick, seemingly doing all the right things. What many people fail to realize is that the invisibles actually count for something. What I mean by the invisibles are the things that we cannot necessarily put our hands on, or see, but yet are just as real as the things that can be seen. If someone came up to you and punched you in the face, just as hard as they could, not only would you be taken by surprise, but you would also, feel the pain associated with the hard blow. Although it came really quick, you still knew at some point that it was coming, even though you did not expect it.

Consider a throbbing headache, how intense the pain and aggravation is to your entire being, yet you cannot see the headache, nor can you really know for sure when it is coming. The point is, just because you cannot predict it or tangibly hold a headache does not diminish its realness. It is just as real as the blow to your face you just can't see it.

The things that you cannot necessarily see can actually eat away at your health little by little, even though you may not recognize it. Before you actually realize it, they have so corroded your soul that you can barely function. After which, those invisible enemies go from one realm, your soul, to your body, and then begins the process of degenerating your health.

Spinal care

No discussion on improving your body's ability to heal would be complete without talking about how

Chiropractic adjustments influence your body's ability to heal. Here again the intangibles have extreme importance. What you cannot feel about Chiropractic care is far more important than what you can.

You can feel the immediate effects of a spinal adjustment from your Chiropractor such as the increase of flexibility and your overall sense of well being. You can see and feel the obvious and immediate improvement in your posture.

Chiropractic care has massive impact on healing ability.

You usually can feel the small popping sound that often accompanies the gentle push of the Chiropractors hands as the spinal bones effortlessly go back into proper position. What you cannot feel is even more important.

We will cover the subject in more detail in other areas of this work so allow me to give you a thumbnail version here. Chiropractic care has massive impact on healing ability. Your spine is the switchboard to your entire body. Nerves emminate from small openings between the twenty four vertebrae that make up the spine. These nerves look and act like electrical wires which carry messages from the brain to the body and back.

When a spinal bone gets shifted out of alignment from birth trauma, a fall, car accident, sports impact, lifting injury, or from muscular tension caused by stress, etc. it irritates the nerve coming out between the vertebrae. The irritation to the nerve interferes or blocks the messages flowing over the nerve similar to how pinching a garden hose blocks the flow of water through the hose. Spinal mis-alignments are a serious health hazard which typically cannot be felt for months or years after the original insult that caused it, sometimes never. That is why regular spinal checkups are so necessary.

Healing in the body is controlled directly by our nerves and the nerve system.

Healing in the body is controlled directly by our nerves and the nerve system. When nerves cannot function normally due to pressure caused by mal-alignment our bodies cannot heal normally. Releasing the pressure on the nerves by regularly checking and realigning the spine insures great healing ability to resume inside. Great healing happening on the inside all of the time means fantastic health. I am fond of saying that "a healthier spine means a healthier you!"

Developing A New Mind

Years ago there was a major slogan, which said, "A Mind Is A Terrible Thing To Waste." This catchphrase was used repeatedly in television commercials, radio announcements, and printed advertisements as a reminder to potential donors, that they could and should financially help, young African-American college-bound students to afford a college education. The whole basis of their appeal is that if people who are blessed to contribute to this worthy cause choose not to, that they would be perpetuating a cyclical crisis of wasting minds.

They will be a part of the problem rather than a solution to the problem without even realizing it. I really like the idea of giving to the mind. Because whatever you deposit into the mind will not only grow with interest, but you will be able to one day make a sizeable withdrawal once your deposit has matured. I wholeheartedly believe in supporting such causes, such as helping young under-priviledged men and women to reach their full God-given potential becoming clear contributors to humanity. I also know that anyone who does not feed and educate their minds will inevitably become a liability to society whether they are black, brown, white, yellow, red, or green.

What you put into your mind is what will come out of it. Great minds do not occur accidentally, it is an intentional effort. Great chiropractors, lawyers, ministers, writers, educators, politicians, activists, and athletes all became great because they decided to and self-disciplined themselves to learn more and work harder than their competition. And because of that they shine above the rest. This same principle applies to the area of health. What you deposit into your mental bank account about health is exactly what you are going to get in return.

Throughout the course of your entire life you have developed a certain mindset and beliefs about your health most often instilled by your parents and teachers. Those beliefs and thought patterns are sometimes difficult to change especially if they have been built on fear, which much of medicine's concepts about health are built on. But they can change once you become aware of them. Let me give you an example. Many people have come to believe that ear infections must be treated with antibiotics to go away. It is now clearly known that treating ear infections with antibiotics is no better than giving the child a pain reliever to relieve the pain and allowing the body three or four days to beat the infection itself. It is also been shown that giving antibiotics may help shut down the infection in the present but actually doubles or triples the likelihood of the infection recurring within two or three weeks. The antibiotics thwart the body's ability to develop antibodies and therefore a permanent immunity to the bad bacteria that is causing the infection. Keeping the child comfortable while allowing the body to work through and

...antibiotics thwart the body's ability to develop antibodies and therefore a permanent immunity to the bad bacteria...

heal the infection is therefore the best approach to dealing with ear infections as well as many other childhood disorders such as fevers, colds and flu.

Medical doctors have difficulty changing their belief systems, too. Regardless of hundreds of research studies, articles and scientific discussions on the topic of the overuse and abuse of antibiotics M.D.'s continue to routinely prescribe antibiotics for ear infections. I am amazed at how often they prescribe antibiotics for viral infections which antibiotics have absolutely no effect upon. Remember the germ theory? Old ideas die hard. Some people would rather hold onto lies rather than change their perspectives. Sometimes it is easier to hold on until the old beliefs than it is to change and embrace the new knowledge and understanding.

Most people, myself included, hate to admit that they are wrong, even when all of the evidence clearly proves them wrong. The first challenge to overcome is the challenge of developing a new mindset about health. So we need to be diligent in educating ourselves realizing that we don't know everything and being willing to accept new evidence and new thinking. There clearly is room for us all to examine and expand our thinking. As a consumer of health care ask many questions of your health providers so that you can make better more informed decisions.

In order to do that, you will have to willingly abandon all of your familial and societal expectations about health. It's those things that have shaped the way you think. In America the average lifespan is about 75 years old. Your relatives may have an extensive history resulting in long battles with cancer, dealing with alcoholism, suffering from heart disease, or diabetes. All of those things may be true, but that does not mean those things are necessarily true for you. Just because America has statistics about the average lifespan does not mean that you have to be average or worse yet below those averages.

You can live a long fruitful life if you change your mind-set. Your family may have a sad history of sickness but you can be the one to break the cycle, defy the odds and set a new course. That will only happen though, when you choose to change your mind about what you should be able to experience in the area of health. Will that be an easy task, particularly since your mind has been the way that it is for so long now? It'll be just as easy as you make it. It probably won't happen overnight, but the process will begin with the very first thought that you choose to change.

Choosing your thoughts

Whether you realize it or not, you have the power to choose the thoughts that you think. Many people falsely believe that they have no control over their thoughts. Nothing could be further from the truth. You have total and complete power over every thought that pops into your mind. You are able to choose your thoughts. Okay, you are probably wondering, how can I choose my thoughts when they just seem to pop up in my mind unexpectedly? You have the power to choose whether you will actually entertain and embrace those thoughts or not. Sickness is a thought. Have you ever heard of sick thoughts? And as long as you choose to entertain sick thoughts you will eventually become the sick thought that you've chosen to ponder.

I once heard of a person that went to the medical doctor's office to get her routine checkup. The doctor examined this lady and went through his normal process of taking tests, drawing blood, and checking her vitals. This lady did not have any fear at all, since she had been a relatively healthy woman and had always received a clean bill of health each time she received a physical. The doctor routinely sent her home, promising to get her the results from her physical within a week's time.

Exactly one week from the date of her physical, the doctor called her at her home expecting to speak with her about his findings. She wasn't at home, so he simply left a message, "This is your Doctor, please call me when you arrive home, I need to talk with you." When she came home, and walked into her room she noticed a blinking light on her phone signaling her that an message was left on the voicemail. She dialed in for her messages, and listened to each one clearly, until she got to the message from her doctor that said, "Please call me."

She quickly returned his call. When the receptionist patched her through to the doctor, he responded in a very somber tone, asking the lady to come in. He told her that he would prefer to not speak about her health on the phone, but rather in a more private setting. His tone appeared somewhat strange to her, he never sounded this way before. She came in right away. Her doctor was not expecting her to make it over to his office as fast as she did, but was quite relieved to know that this uncomfortable announcement would not have to be prolonged and that his meeting with her would not last very long.

He told her that the tests that were taken proved that she was infected with the AIDS virus, and that it was so far gone, that she would not live more than a few months. Immediately she began crying hysterically. Being in her early thirties she could not understand why this was all happening to her. She could not think of a legitimate cause for the disease particularly since she was not a promiscuous woman. As a nurse she had been stuck with needles on several occasions after injecting sickened patients. She immediately connected her contracting AIDS to that. She thanked the doctor for his honest communication and left stunned.

Over the next several days, this woman began to embrace her illness and began to associate every negative reaction and symptom she felt to the virus, seemingly trying her best to demonstrate each one. She began to lose weight, going from 135 pounds to less than 80 pounds. She actually developed lesions on her flesh. The following week, she woke up one morning and began to vomit blood. When she went to comb her hair, a patch of hair fell into the sink. This wonderful woman had been pitifully convinced that the doctor's estimation of several months was really far less, and she was mentally preparing to die.

Her health had failed so miserably low, that it was quite obvious that she probably would not live for another week, unless some sort of divine intervention took place. One day while she was coughing and feeling totally sick all over, her phone rang. It was her doctor, far more chipper this time, asking her to come in. At this point she had already conceded to die, and really did not want to hear anymore negative news, as she had suffered enough already. Honoring the long-standing relationship that she had with her doctor, she went at his request.

When she arrived, far slower than she did when she first went, she found her doctor sporting a huge smile on his face. At first she almost felt a bit offended. "Why would anyone be smiling at such a time? I am going to die any minute now, and he thinks that's a reason to smile," she thought. Her doctor told her that I have good news and bad news. The bad news is that I made a mistake with regard to my diagnosis of your condition and I have not been as accurate as I should be with my information.

The good news though, is that I switched your test results with another patient. You do not have AIDS at all. You have a perfectly clean bill of health. At first, the woman did not know how to respond. For the past three weeks she had acted out on the thoughts that she kept pondering. She thought that she was supposed to act like a dying woman, so she did. And even though she was not physically sick at all, her powerful negative thoughts actually produced the same type of results as if she were genuinely ill with the disease.

Your thoughts have the potential to produce very negative or very positive results.

The other person whose file was switched with hers, the woman that actually had the disease, never faltered a bit in her health. She did not vomit, lose hair, contract a high fever, or break out in lesions. The reason is because she did not have any negative thoughts to feed on. What a powerful example!

Do you see how powerful your thoughts are and just how sick you can become if you continue to act on sickly thoughts? Your thoughts have the potential to produce very negative or very positive results. Think healthy thoughts. If you think healthy thoughts then you will invariably reap the benefits from those thoughts. Conversely, if you constantly think death and disease, surely, in time those thoughts can become your reality.

My friend and mentor Bob Harrison says that we always move toward our most dominant thoughts and pictures that we hold in our mind. We tend to get exactly what we expect in life. Change what you are thinking about and expecting and watch your life move toward it over time.

Watch What You Say

In the most literal sense your words create your world. Really, the amount of money that you have or do not have can be directly connected to the words you speak about money. You probably don't think that deeply about it but it's really true. If you continue to say things like, "I'm broke, I don't have any money, I can't afford that" then you will continue to live in lack since our words create our experience.

I am very careful about the words that I speak. Because I am such an advocate of great health, I don't even jokingly play games about my health using stupid phrases such as, "I know I'm gonna get sick, or I always get sick when, or no one in my family ever had good health." I never say things even close to these, because I know that when I do it sets a very negative wheel in motion.

Since I do not want sickness, I do not speak about sickness. I only voice the things that I desire. I speak the things that I expect to have, expect to own, and expect to enjoy in life. Anything else, does not qualify to come out of my mouth. Now I realize that that requires huge self-discipline for most people, especially those people that say anything that comes to mind without first thinking about their consequences. Begin now to keep from voicing those negative thoughts that keep popping into your head and replace them with positive ones. You may say that is easier said than done and that may be true in the beginning. I know that firsthand but nothing great ever came without some hard work first. Health consciousness is a lifestyle. Begin believing that bad health is no longer an option. Start speaking and expecting only the best for your future.

Great health belongs to any person that chooses to go after it.

Great health belongs to any person that chooses to go after it. If you are that kind of person, and I suspect that you are, you will welcome change, knowing that change is good and rewarding. So I want you to begin saying out loud everyday, "I am thankful for my great health, I look forward to living a long, healthy life, thank you God for answering my prayers and healing my body, I expect to be well my whole life long, my health gets better everyday, my cholesterol is normal, I am disease-free," etc. You need to begin speaking like that. Keep saying it until it becomes real to you.

Saying it aloud helps your subconscious mind to act on it. I am not sure exactly how or why it works but I know it does work. How will you know that it is real and that it is working? You will know as you see your health improving and your attitudes about your health changing. You will know it is working when you begin hearing yourself telling others to watch what they say, teaching others the other concepts you are learning by reading this book and when you no longer consider bad health an option.

> *You become a chained slave to anyone you choose not to forgive....*
>
> ～

Forgiveness

This may sound a bit strange but people can get extremely ill when they choose to harbor feelings of bitterness and resentment inside of them. This is not a Sunday school lesson but rather a lesson that so many millions of people neglect and as a result end up living a life half of what they could or should actually enjoy. Throughout the course of my life, I have had people do things to me that were wrong, but I choose to forgive them. You become a chained slave to anyone you choose not to forgive even when they were completely in the wrong.

The reason why I so readily forgive them is not for them as much as it is for me. I forgive them because I do not want to live with the negativity associated with their terrible actions. Whatever you are not willing to release inevitably stays with you, not with them. And as it stays with you, it will never stay in its original state, but continue to fester and grow larger and larger until it has overtaken you. When you don't forgive other people, it's not only a spiritual or mental concern, but also is a huge health concern.

If you are not careful these events can become defining moments that you get stuck in for the rest of your life. It can also become an excuse for everything you never accomplished in your life from that point forward. You know within five minutes when you are speaking to someone that has allowed this to happen. It doesn't take long before you hear about the horrible divorce they went through, their wretched ex-spouse, or the drunk driver that ripped the heart from their chest when they killed their child and changed everything. I am not saying their hurt is not legitimate. I am saying that we have choices to get bitter or get better. Choose to get better.

I know that people who harbor resentment within them often develop ulcers, cancer, suffer strokes, and heart attacks as a direct result. Imagine an eighteen-wheeler truck trying to navigate around on a set of Toyota Camry tires and wheels. Even if you could trick out an eighteen wheeler to look good that way, those small tires would blow out moments after the truck took off down the road and hit a few small bumps. The tires would quickly become destroyed since they are carrying more weight than they are designed to carry.

You are no different. You were not designed to carry unnecessary garbage and unwarranted weight on your shoulders. There are more than enough things in life that you already have to deal with, without having to add the stress of unforgiveness, bitterness, regret, jealousy, or envy. Don't carry anyone else's evilness around inside you. When you do that it becomes yours and slowly eats away at you on the inside until you have a major blowout. Release it, release them, set yourself free and live!

What You Hear

I've talked a bit about the words that come out of your mouth and the affects that it can have on you. You should also be very careful about the words that you allow others to speak around you. You cannot afford to listen to just everything. Everything that you hear has a major impact on your life. Don't listen to gossip. You ask, "What does that have to do with good health?" It has everything to do with good health.

Gossip is essentially the process of tearing others down. When you use your mouth to tear others down, you are tearing yourself down in the process. If you use your tongue to build others up, then you will be strong and built up also. Some people believe that they can listen to others tear people down, and as long as they don't join in, it's all right. Not so. Listening to other people's negative chatter is almost as bad for you as doing it yourself.

None of us can afford negative thinking.

~

Your silence can often be taken as a sign that you are consenting to what they are saying. So it's better not to hear it at all. If you have friends or family members that have a bad habit of always complaining or talking about sickness, lack or frequently talking about how the family is known to suffer from this disease or that sickness, you may have to correct them. If they do not respond appropriately you may have to quarantine yourself away from them for a season. Negative speech corrupts thought and negative thought affects actions and influences character. Negativity definitely affects health. None of us can afford negative thinking.

In the same way that you guard who watches your children and who you allow to come into your home you should guard the words and music that you listen to. Your health is your most valuable personal asset and it is worth going to extremes to protect it.

Fasting

In nearly every world religion, fasting is a valued practice used not only for spiritual and self discipline reasons but also as a bodily cleansing agent. Fasting in its most literal sense is abstaining from food. But the purpose in doing so is not to give rise to starvation to lose weight. As we discussed earlier fasting to lose weight is a bad strategy.

Fasting gives your insides a much-needed rest.

∼

Fasting has many tremendous benefits, but I'll highlight just a few. One of the main things that fasting does is it detoxifies your body. That means that while you are fasting your body goes through a process of ridding itself of harmful toxins that ultimately hinder good health.

Most people are totally shocked when they realize just how toxic their bodies are. The average person is full of poisons from medication usage, environmental pollution, pesticides, etc. and don't even realize it. Whatever you eat , breathe or drink works it way into your blood system and into your tissues causing your entire body to become vulnerable to disease and distress. That is why making healthier food and beverage choices is so important. When you fast, in a sense it is like resting your insides which helps it to clean itself up and enables it to work at more optimal levels.

Fasting gives your insides a much-needed rest. We live in a consumer and stress-filled world, and food is perhaps the most consumed commodity of all. People eat all of the time, seemingly non-stop often in reaction to stress. When you wake up, you eat breakfast. Then in between breakfast and lunch, you've probably had a snack or two. After eating lunch, a candy bar and soda in the mid afternoon. Then an enormous dinner and late at night a beverage or nightcap or two with more munchies. The bottom line is that your digestive system is always working hard and never able to get much rest. Anything that does not get the rest that it needs, will tire and begin working inefficiently from over exhaustion.

If you drove your car from my hometown in Hershey, Pennsylvania to Washington State nonstop, only pulling over to get gas, yet never turned the car off, your car might easily overheat because it is being overworked. Work horses, and oxen that pull heavy loads both require rest, too.

You have a car or two in your garage but my Amish patients have a horse and buggy in theirs. After driving their horse and carriage fifteen or twenty miles to visit with family or friends they must rest their horse for several hours before they can drive him back home. In the hot summer months they stop and hose them down to cool them off and give them water at a friends home along the way.

The digital printing presses that printed this book have an unbelievable capacity to print thousands of sheets each hour and can run for hours at a time. But even high-tech sophisticated machinery has to get a break every now and then for repairs and maintenance. You can run machinery all day long, pretty much non-stop. But when you do that you increase the probability of something going wrong and increasing the likelihood of needing repairs.

Your digestive track needs time to rest for the same reason that the rest of your body does, so it can have energy to complete its daily tasks without faltering. When you fast, you give your digestive system the break it desperately needs.

At certain times my wife and I will fast one day a week for a month or two for spiritual reasons as well as for health and weight management motivations. You can too.

Experts discourage late night eating for the same reasons to give your digestive track a break overnight. When you go to sleep your digestive tract should go to sleep with you. One of the main reasons why people feel fatigued and tired when they wake in the morning, is because they eat so late. Then when their bodies are supposed to be sleeping, their digestive tract is steadily working the night shift from 11 PM to 6 AM, working diligently to digest food.

SETTING THINGS STRAIGHT

Have you ever noticed that heavy roadwork on major highways is often done late at night, while you are sleeping? The reason why they choose the late night hours is because, they know that the traffic is minimal and that they won't have to worry about anything obstructive getting in their way while they work. You can apply the same concept to your body. There are certain things that can only get fixed in your body when your body takes a rest from food.

My wife and I have this discussion often about how interesting it is that God made us and most all living things to need a time each day for refreshing and restoration. Sleep is really sort of a weird thing if you stop and think about it. Our bodies go into a strange almost coma-like state. Sleep gives the body a break and a chance to rebuild, repair and rejuvenate itself. Eating too late interrupts the natural cycles of sleep and therefore robs the body of much needed healing and rebooting time. People that don't sleep well are typically poor healers for that reason.

Many cancer patients at the Oasis Clinic in Mexico have been totally cured from cancer. One of their many natural healing methods is fasting. They put many of their new patients through a fasting process to aid in detoxification. After that they begin to feed the body only very nutrient rich foods that help it to repair and rebuild itself from the inside out.

As you can see the intangibles are as important as the things we can see and feel. You can't see a fast; neither can you see what is going on inside of you. However, you do know when you are fasting because you immediately feel the hunger associated with fasting. Do your best to overcome the affects of the hunger and give rise to your body's natural ability to heal itself. You can cut the affects of hunger by drinking 4-6 ounces of natural, no sugar added juice every couple of hours. Some would argue with me but I find grapefruit juice works well for me personally. When I fast I usually do it for three days at a time with water and juices only. Drink plenty of pure water, which helps your liver, kidneys and lymphatic system to purge themselves of impurities and toxins. Once I get past the first day I have little to no hunger or desire for food. You will be amazed how clearly you will think and how much of your day revolves around preparing, thinking about, eating and cleaning up food.

CHAPTER SIX

The Non-Drug Approach To Lowering Your Cholesterol

If you have ever been diagnosed with high cholesterol I would hope that your doctor gave you a brief education about what cholesterol is and how it works in your body however I cannot assume that. If you haven't had that lesson, allow me to briefly inform you about this subject. Cholesterol is not bad for you as some people falsely assume. In fact, your body needs cholesterol and lots of it. Your body requires it to produce hormones, restore cell membranes, and to process vitamin D. Your brain and nerve system are full of it and in fact requires it to work properly. This is why the no cholesterol, no fat diet fad has created serious problems for some people.

I am just not convinced that cholesterol and all the hype surrounding it is the big deal that the medical and pharmaceutical industry say that it is. These two industries make billions per year and stand to gain the most from creating a new disease craze and all of the fear factors that go with it. How else can you explain that just a few years ago normal blood cholesterol was considered to be 220. Now it has been lowered to 200 and there is talk of moving it to 180. Every step down encircles a vast increase of millions of people who can be scared into taking anti-cholesterol medications along with all the accoutrements of additional doctors' visits, blood tests, etc. It all adds up to big business for doctors, hospitals and drug companies and don't be fooled by it.

The problem occurs whenever cholesterol levels get too high because it can heighten the risk of heart disease, heart attack and stroke. The major concern is build up in the arteries of the heart and blood vessels which is a condition called atherosclerosis. For the average person, your cholesterol level should be somewhere in the area of 200. When your cholesterol exceeds 240 there is room for concern so it is important to keep your cholesterol level in the normal range definitely below this to avoid heart, brain and blood vessel damage.

My professional and personal comfort level is 220 or below. I believe that prescribing medication for anything under 240 is ridiculous. The problem as I see it is that drugs are the easy way out. It is always best to look at natural ways to manage cholesterol levels first. Weight loss, increasing aerobic exercise and nutritional supplements are the first things to consider. Then and only after needed weight loss has occurred, intense exercise and appropriate dietary changes have been made and failed to produce results should medication be considered.

When a person has discovered that their cholesterol is high, too often people seek prescription-based solutions to help lower their cholesterol levels because television marketing has conditioned the general public to do so. Drug marketing definitely works. Although most

Cholesterol medications can have major side effects.

doctors would gladly write a prescription for you, what most of them do not realize is that there are many proven alternatives to lower your cholesterol levels other than drugs. Cholesterol medications can have major side effects. Those so called side effects can in some cases cause permanent damage to organs and cause death so you must take every drug recommendation seriously.

I've always considered it a pretty bad exchange or even a bad deal to get one benefit yet lose another in the process that may be of far greater value. Don't lose your arm to get a leg. You need both your arm and your leg to function optimally. Side effects of cholesterol medication are serious. Here are a few scary ones right off the fine print in a magazine drug advertisement for one of the most popular anti-cholesterol drugs. They are liver cancer, cirrhosis of the liver, liver failure, impotency (the inability to achieve erection), autoimmune disease (a condition where the body produces antibodies against itself) and psychotic disturbances to name just a few. I believe that the bad effects of cholesterol drugs themselves and even the supposed good effects of the drugs long term are worse than the potential effects of having mild to moderately high cholesterol levels. I am aware there are many that would disagree with me on this point.

So I've dedicated this section to giving you some alternatives to aid yourself in the process of bringing your cholesterol level to where it needs to be. I'll recommend some vitamins that help to increase the healthy function of the liver and can also help to reduce your cholesterol levels.

I'll also suggest some foods to eat and some foods that you should probably stay away from since they have a high concentration of cholesterol. However, changing your diet alone will not always do the trick. It's usually a combination of many things working together that will work for you. Only about twenty percent of your cholesterol comes from your diet. The other eighty percent comes from your liver.

That does not mean that you can eat anything that you choose to and expect to be healthy. Diet may represent twenty percent of your cholesterol intake, but if your liver is already producing the sufficient amounts for your body, the 20 % that comes from foods can push you over the top, putting you in a high risk category, the place you don't want to be.

Foods To Eat

As you already know I do not recommend dieting, as most people understand it. However, I do believe that you should adjust your eating habits, slowly but surely, adding certain foods to your meal plan and taking some away. In many cases dieting can have the same negative results as taking pills. There are certain diets that are low fat, no fat and low carb diets that may help you to lose weight, but may also have adverse reactions that can be deadly. Don't look for the quick fix or the miracle diet.

Simply make some small changes and build on each change that you've made until you recognize the larger results within you. Here are some foods that help to ward off bad cholesterol in your body and also help to lower your cholesterol in general. Understand, that it is not just eating these foods once in a lifetime that will produce results; rather it's when you incorporate them into your overall day to day lifestyle that you will begin to feel better and experience an improvement in your cholesterol levels and in your health.

- Fish—Try to increase your fish intake of farm-raised fish to two to three times each week. Fish like trout, salmon, halibut, and perch are especially good for you. Fish meat is high in Omega 3 oils known to be very helpful with cholesterol lowering and is anti-inflammatory. I am recommending farm or deep, cold water fish due to high mercury levels found in so many other fish. When preparing the fish try to bake it, grill or broil it. Stay away from fried foods of any kind, as it tends to increase your cholesterol levels. Also stay away from catfish, and shellfish such as lobster, crabs, and shrimp, all of which can increase your cholesterol levels also. These guys are primarily bottom feeders which makes them generally not a good food source. Some people falsely believe that all seafood is equally good for you. Not so, some seafood can be just as harmful to your body as certain meats. Just because you have a seafood only diet does not mean that you are home free. It depends on the seafood, where it comes from and how you prepare it.

- Whole Grain—Whether pasta or bread products, transition from white starchy products to whole grain. For the most part, white food products, particularly breads and pasta, are refined and processed food products and are typically bleached. That's how it gets its white color. They usually have little to no nutritional value, as its nutrients get stripped in the processing. You can generally request whole grain products at most fine restaurants and most grocery stores carry many whole grain breads and pastas. They may cost slightly more than their white counterparts, but are much healthier. Check the labels, however, and choose the most natural choices possible.

- Oatmeal—Within the past decade there has been quite a bit of concentration on the many benefits of oatmeal. In recent years the FDA actually gave its consent to label oatmeal as a food that helps to prevent heart disease. Obviously, that truth is not a new find. Oatmeal has always been a great food, low in fat, high in fiber, and very delicious. I recommend it as a very good choice for breakfast. Fiber gives you favor with cholesterol. At least one study has shown that adding oatmeal to your diet can lower cholesterol levels by 40% due mostly to its high fiber content. Try adding nuts, ground flax seed and/or stevia (natural sweetener) to add variety.

- Green Vegetables, especially green leafy vegetables—Your mom told you about this one, years ago. I am here to remind you again. Eat more vegetables! Mama was right! Vegetables are low-carb, low calorie, high fiber, and extremely healthy for you. It's one of the few things that you can eat as much as you'd like and not have to worry about gaining weight. The more raw and steamed vegetables you eat the better. Don't overcook your vegetables. When you do they will lose the vitamins, minerals, and enzymes and fiber which ultimately defeats the whole purpose. Here is a small list of proven vegetables that increases your healthy heart function and specifically been shown to lower cholesterol: Spinach, lettuce, green beans, cabbage, broccoli, turnip greens, and mustard greens.

- Olive Oil and Walnut Oil—All oils are not necessarily good for you. Stay clear of vegetable shortening, cheap oils and pork products. When you purchase olive oil, stick with extra virgin olive oil. It costs more than most oils, but is worth every dime. Extra Virgin Olive Oil simply means that it is the purest and most natural form of olive oil that you can purchase.

- Fiber—Adding extra fiber in your diet is my number two best anti-cholesterol strategy second to taking organic flaxseed oil 1-2 tablespoons per day. You can find fiber drinks at many health food stores, which often contain psyllium and/or ground flax seed. Fiber makes the bowels move faster pulling along with it toxins, reducing constipation and decreasing a disorder called leaky gut syndrome. You can add ground flax seeds on salads and in homemade breads and healthy muffins, too.

- Eat Fresh Fruits including strawberries, blueberries, and blackberries.

- New research has discovered that these foods have been found also to have a lowering effect on cholesterol levels: Garlic, shiitake mushrooms, avocados, almonds, soy beans, pinto beans, navy beans, kidney beans, onions, and red hot chili peppers.

What's Eating At You?

Quite obviously you should avoid any food that is proven to increase your cholesterol. I know it can be hard but try to limit eating rich, fattening desserts. They taste good, but there is a high price to pay after you've eaten them. Choose fruits instead or go without. If you just have to have the banana cream pie or coconut custard pie, try not to eat it as often as you have been. If you typically have desserts every day or even five times a week, cut your dessert intake in half. Have dessert only twice a week instead. Remember every little bit counts.

It's time for true confessions from a converted and reformed sugar-holic. One of my favorite desserts (and still is) is the world famous Hershey's Chocolate Cream Pie served at none other than the four star Hotel Hershey in Hershey, Pennsylvania, the chocolate capital of the world. The main street here is Chocolate Avenue. Even the streetlights are shaped like Hershey's Kisses. Having been born and raised here it seems unlikely that I would have become such a strong natural health advocate, doesn't it? I was doomed to sugarholism right from the start.

Most peanut butters are made out of partially hydrogenated oil....

~

I have eliminated all the bad stuff from my diet but I do still enjoy a few bites of chocolate cream pie or New York Style cheesecake when I am out for a nice dinner. I have learned that I can get all the enjoyment without the detriment by just eating a few bites and passing the rest around the table for others to enjoy, too.

Avoid all foods that are high in saturated fat. Saturated fat comes from animal foods such as pork, beef, dairy products, butter, and cheese, which incidentally tend to be very fattening. Add to the list, any and all processed foods. Generally anything that is packaged has been processed and has high contents of saturated fat and bad oils. Coconut oil, palm oil, and even cocoa butter are all high in saturated fat. Trash the French fries, the margarine, all hydrogenated or partially hydrogenated oils (trans fats), cookies, vegetable shortening, crackers, and yes, potato chips. Most peanut butters are made out of partially hydrogenated oil, peanuts, salt, and mucho sugar so dump it too. All of these can raise your cholesterol and triglyceride levels and can incite pain and inflammation in your body.

Not only can food choices raise your cholesterol but also physical inactivity. When you don't exercise it raises your LDL and lowers your HDL. LDL is an acronym that stands for low density lipoproteins. They are made of fat with very small amounts of protein. This kind of cholesterol is commonly called bad cholesterol because it clogs your arteries. HDL stands for high density lipoproteins and is commonly referred to as good cholesterol.

Being overweight raises your triglycerides and lowers your good cholesterol (HDL). Having a sluggish thyroid can also raise cholesterol levels. Smoking is very counterproductive to your health, partly because your HDL is lowered when you smoke worsening your overall health. Please be mindful of that.

You need to know where you stand, in terms of your overall health. This is why I encourage you to have a Chiropractor, a natural-minded M.D. (they do exist), naturopath and other natural health care providers as part of your family's health team. Other natural disciplines to definitely consider would be homeopaths, nutrition specialists, massage therapy, reflexology, colon hydrotherapy, and acupuncture. Natural health care providers generally have a much broader understanding of how to help the body function better without resorting to drastic, riskier medical treatments which can always be used as a last resort.

Here is a good way to know where your cholesterol levels are. I've provided below a list to show you where your cholesterol and your LDL should be. So the objective is to lower your LDL and increase your HDL. The truth is that if you follow the recommendations I have laid out for you throughout this book, most of this takes care of itself.

Total cholesterol—less than 200 (mg/dL)

Borderline High—in between 200-239

High Cholesterol—240 or higher

Perfect LDL—below 100 (mg/dL)

Good LDL—in between 100-129

Borderline High LDL—in between 130-159

High LDL—in between 160-189

Too High LDL—190 or higher

The Dream Team—Vitamins & Supplements

One of the wonderful things about health research is that people are finding out more discoveries than ever before that will help you to lower your cholesterol naturally. This list is not a comprehensive list. It is, however, a great starting point.

- Omega 3 Oil—Omega has become very popular within the past five years or so. It comes from fish oil and flax seed oil. It is also very helpful in reducing inflammation in the body, which can be a major risk factor for cardiovascular disease. This is my number one dietary recommendation for lowering cholesterol. I recommend that all of my adult patients take one to two tablespoons of flax seed oil per day. A side benefit is that it naturally relieves pain and inflammation in the body. It is especially helpful for those with arthritis, Fibromyalgia, Chronic Fatigue Syndrome, and any other multiple joint pain problems.

- Garlic—Legend has it that garlic is known for keeping vampires away. That has never been proven. It has been proven that garlic reduces cholesterol though many forms of garlic in pill form have a very strong aftertaste and odor. They do have pill forms of odorless garlic available. Cook with fresh garlic as often as possible.

- Niacin— is one form of vitamin B. I suggest that you take a relatively large dose of natural, not synthetic, B complex vitamin daily. This is great advice for all kinds of issues. It helps those who crave sugar, have joint problems, fight anxiety, and depression. I have seen many cases of anxiety and panic attacks be caused by vitamin B deficiency. Niacin specifically has been shown to help lower cholesterol.

- Chromium-GTF—is mostly known for aiding sugar metabolism and blood sugar levels. It can also be very instrumental in lowering cholesterol.

- Octacosanol—is from wheat germ oil. It can lower cholesterol.

- Beta-carotene—Carotene is fat-soluble orange pigment found in green leafy vegetables, and also in carrots, tomatoes, pumpkins, and mangoes. It is absorbed through the small intestine walls where it is converted into vitamin A. It promotes good vision and healthy skin. In addition to helping to lower cholesterol beta-carotene has properties which guard against certain kinds of cancer, typically lung and cervical cancer. It also helps to protect the eyes and skin from ultraviolet rays from the sun.

If you want to get the maximum benefit from any of these supplements, follow carefully the instructions on the labels. Ask your Chiropractor or other natural health care provider to assist you in knowing what to take and in what doses.

CHAPTER SEVEN

Diabetes—Prevention and Control

⎯⎯⦿⎯⎯

According to the American Diabetes Association there are 20.8 million adults and children in the United States that have diabetes. This means that 7% of the entire population has this disease. Of this 20.8 million person figure, 14.6 million people have been diagnosed with diabetes, the other 6.2 million are living with diabetes yet do not realize it. Added to that, 41 million people are in a pre-diabetes stage. For them, it is just a matter of time before the effects of the disease actually manifest. Diabetes is one of the fastest growing diseases with 1.5 million new adult cases in 2005 alone.

In 2002, there were 224,092 documented deaths that were directly connected to this illness. This figure is really far more than that, particularly in older persons that suffer with diabetes that worsened other chronic health problems such as heart disease and high blood pressure. The costs are staggering as well. In 2002 alone the total annual economic costs of diabetes was low-balled around $132 billion. That grandiose figure represents 1 out of every 10 health care dollars spent in the United States of America.[1]

The facts prove that diabetes is big business and the drug and medical industries are in no hurry to see it go away. If you owned, operated or shared in a business that raked in $132 billion in revenues annually, how quickly would you want to shut it down? Okay, I know the answer. You would never want to shut it down. And the reasons are very obvious. No one in their right mind shuts down a business that is extremely lucrative. They may sell them or merge them with another corporation, but they never want to shut them down. Just let the money keep on streaming in. Like so many other diseases a cure would mean loss of huge revenue so they are not quick to encourage you to fix or find other alternatives for your disease or condition. They can easily rationalize their reasons for doing so.

You have been totally lied to concerning diabetes for years. You've been lied to for so long that you actually

---

1. *Source: American Diabetes Association*
   http://www.diabetes.org/diabetes-statistics.jsp

believe that the lies that you've been brainwashed with are actually true. The main lie that you've been fed is that there is no cure for diabetes or no natural way of helping it. They also have told you that there is nothing that you can do by yourself for yourself and that you will just have to live with the disease, forever. That's a big fat lie. I can get very upset about this topic especially when innocent people get hurt. I hate it when the medical and pharmaceutical industries collaborate together to get and keep you ignorant of the wide and varied choices that you have concerning your health. They claim to have your best interest in mind but do not think for a minute that they are not in bed with one another. They stand to lose a ton of money and power when you start thinking for yourself and taking a more active role in your health.

> *They stand to lose a ton of money and power when you start thinking for yourself and taking a more active role in your health.*
> ~

I started my personal quest for natural health and wellness 33 years ago. In that timeframe I have been sick two times bad enough that I sought the help of a medical doctor. In thirty three years I have needed the help of a prescription medicine one time for ten days. I have been sick other times but only with minor colds and sore throats but have always cared for them naturally with Chiropractic adjustments, vitamins, plant extracts, herbs and/or rest. This book is really about the way I live my life and think and care for my own family and my patients. Needless to say the medical doctors and drug companies have not made much income from me, my family or my patients for that matter. Wellness works. Sickness is expensive. Disease is lucrative.

Diabetes is nearly always preventable, sometimes curable, and always treatable.

The number one reason that the drug and medical profession has sold you on this lie is because of money. Money is a great motivator. It is the impetus that causes divorces, friendships to be destroyed, businesses like Enron to go sour, and even multiple millions of people to suffer mercilessly and die each year without a hope. I'm here to tell you that you do have options. Diabetes is nearly always preventable, sometimes curable and always treatable. Many cases of diabetes can be addressed totally naturally without a kitchen tabletop full of deadly drugs, many of which carry a heavy price when used long term. Let's face it; if you get cured from diabetes, they'll have lost a valuable customer.

They want your business; because they know that your business is extremely profitable for them. Beyond that, they don't want you to know that you have other possible options. It's the same way with other chronic and supposedly incurable diseases like cancer and arthritis. Be prepared when you decide that you no longer want to use the myriad of drugs that the doctor prescribed for you to take for the rest of your life.

When you decide that you really want to use a more natural approach and natural alternatives, they immediately start spewing out a whole lot of scare tactics. I've known of countless situations when medical doctors actually told my patients that they were going to die if they did not take the drugs. It is a control issue and they use fear to control you. It heightens when you threaten to go against

When you decide to divest out of this profitable system you have declared a war, whether you realize it or not.

their authority especially when they know that you want to tap into and explore a different method of healing.

It gets worse. I have on multiple occasions had medical doctors tell my patients that they would die if they continued with Chiropractic care. Chiropractors laugh out loud at these types of outrageous statements especially from medical doctors who have admittedly killed hundreds and hundreds of thousand, and harmed millions more over just this last decade alone. Be sure of this: medicine is big business and people die everyday as a result.

My purpose here is not only to give you options in dealing with diabetes or other health problems, nor is it simply to expose the age-old lies that they have been telling you, but my purpose is also to give you a defense mechanism on how to deal with the major pressure that you will receive from the medical profession and society in general when

Decide once and for all that no one in this world is going to take away your right to be healthy, whole and happy.

you make the quality decision to take your health into your own hands. I want to be straightforward with you. When you decide to divest out of this profitable system you have declared a war, whether you realize it or not.

And as with most wars, blood will be shed and people will continue to die before the victory is won. Fortunately for you, many other people have already jumped overboard off the big ship called medicine over the past thirty years. They became wellness pioneers declaring their own health independence.

The world of health care is not flat. The world of wellness and taking responsibility for one's own health is round and many others like myself have proven that life is better across the sea without the drugs, the fear, and the attitude.

Many within my own profession have paid dearly. Many Chiropractors were imprisoned for their beliefs.

Many more like myself have paid and continue to pay huge prices politically, socially and financially so that you won't have to. All you have to do is be prepared for the mind games that they will play on you. This is your life and you need to live it to the max. Decide once and for all that no one in this world is going to take away your right to be healthy, whole and happy. Anyone that attempts to steal those liberties from you should be viewed as the enemy and be avoided at all cost.

Possible Causes

...realize that your body was designed to heal itself....

~

If you suffer with diabetes then I believe that you are pretty likely to know what it actually is. You may not have been diagnosed with the disease but have an interest about it or perhaps people in your bloodline have suffered with diabetes. At any rate being sufficiently armed with knowledge will put you in the winner's seat. Diabetes is a condition that originates when there is an absolute or relative lack of the hormone insulin in the body.

When that happens it produces abnormal variations in the way cells utilize sugar in your body. This is characterized by unusually high levels of sugar in the bloodstream and that is serious. Although juvenile diabetes is growing rapidly in the United States, it is still far higher in obese people and older adults. Although it has been said that there is no cure, realize that your body was designed to heal itself. If you get Chiropractic adjustments, eat right, exercise, and maintain a positive mental attitude, it will automatically attempt to fix and regulate itself when given the chance...always.

So before we can effectively prevent or fix the problem let's first look at some possible reasons people get diabetes to begin with. One of the reasons can be heredity but this sometimes becomes an excuse. The reason that I said excuse is because people tend to think that an excuse releases them from the responsible action they need to take in any given situation. Let's just deal with that one for a moment. The basic idea is that if your mother and father or your siblings suffered with diabetes that you inevitably will also. Not so!

The only way that you are guaranteed to inherit the same types of diseases and sicknesses from your parents and ancestors is if you do the same things that they did, think the way they thought, ate the same way they ate, practiced the same habits and adopted all of the same cultural practices. There are so many contributing factors to the theory of genetically caused diseases. For the most part the predominant assumption is that you have adopted the same genetic traits and habits of your parents.

It is assumed that you have the same eating habits, lack of physical activity, and even stress levels associated with your culture. For example, in African Americans the risk for diabetes is proportionately higher than in European Americans. Incidences in African Americans are second only to Native Americans. That has nothing to do with pre-disposition. That thought is foolishness! Americans of African descent are no more predisposed to become diabetics than Americans of European descent are predisposed to become winners of the PGA tour. The reason why diabetes is higher in African Americans is because of the culture.

In Mediterranean countries...their health is generally far better.

~

African Americans tend to eat foods that are high in fat, salt and other high-sodium seasonings that promote hypertension and heart disease. Sugar and trans fats are also a major part of their diet. I have to admit that African American cooking tastes pretty darn good. That's the good side, great taste. The down side is that this diet over an extended period of time will eventually kill you or anyone else. Collard greens with ham-hocks, macaroni and cheese, barbecue spare ribs, corn bread, good ole sweet candied yams, and Kool-Aid to wash it all down, is a typical Sunday meal for many African American people. It's a cultural thing. Many European American people especially in the southern region of the United States deal with the same problem of diabetes and heart disease for the same reasons.

If you travel to Mediterranean countries, you will find that their culture suggests a totally different kind of diet and consequently their health is generally far better. They eat a lot of olive oil, fresh vegetables, and freshfish. As a result, the incidences of diabetes are far less. In India most of the people there are vegetarians. Native Asians have little incidence of weight, heart or diabetic problems until they come to America and adopt our health habits. In time their disease statistics are exactly the same as ours. So you see that having great health is a decision, not genes or rocket science.

The point is, that if your culture does things that lean toward diabetes, then you have to make a decision not to eat the things that eventually produce that adverse result. You should at least limit your intake. I've said before that moderation is the key. You won't die prematurely, just because you have a real "down home meal" once in a while or develop diabetes if you enjoy a piece of pineapple upside-down cake occasionally.

However, if you eat that way every single day, you will eventually suffer with severe illness and obesity. So when we speak of genetics it's not an automatic thing. In some cases, genetics is a choice based on the decisions that you make to change or alter your cultural habits and create new ones.

The absolute biggest cause of diabetes is the consumption of soda. There are nine teaspoons of sugar in the average twelve ounce can. All that sugar one or more times a day severely stresses and overtaxes your pancreas, the organ that produces insulin and controls your blood sugar. It also packs on the pounds. Diabetes is almost unheard of in people who are normal weight. The second largest cause is inactivity. Therefore weight control and exercise are the two best ways to prevent, cure, and help control diabetes.

> *The absolute biggest cause of diabetes is the consumption of soda.*
>
> ∼

Here are the top reasons why people get diabetes.

Core Reasons:

- Massive Consumption of Soda

- Obesity—(nearly two thirds of Americans are overweight, and most diabetics are overweight)

- Overeating —(nearly 30% of the North American population suffers with an overeating disorder)

- Physical Inactivity/Lack of Exercise (exercise burns calories and is huge key in helping to regulate blood sugar)

- Eating Too Much Sugar, highly processed foods, and carbohydrates

- Excessive Intake of Animal Fats which digest down—(read the sign below the arches, "billions and billions served." We consume far too many animal products.

- Excess Intake of Foods Containing Bad or Low Quality Oils

- Large Portions (diabetics must control portions and make healthier food choices)

- Lack of Self Discipline (making poor food choices by not placing high enough priority on one's own health)

- Stress, Worry, and Unhealthy Grieving—(stress has been linked to mental and physical health problems... More than $300 billion is spent on stress-related compensation claims, absenteeism, insurance costs, and low productivity)

- Hereditary factors—(people tend to mirror the behavioral habits of their parents, whether those habits are good or bad)

If you deal with or eliminate all of these areas or the ones that you most likely have issues with, you will begin to see an immediate improvement in your health. The concept is pretty elementary, just stop doing what you have been doing wrong and you will get favorable results. I know that it may be difficult for you to discipline yourself in an area that you've allowed to get out of control. It'll take a lot of work. My encouragement to you is not to do everything at once. Take one step at a time and you'll be amazed at the results over time.

In my profession in Chiropractic, health maintenance and prevention are paramount. That is one of the many reasons why I love what I do. Despite conventional thinking that waits to fix problems only after they have developed; Chiropractors choose to prevent problems so that they never start in the first place. I would rather prevent trouble than fight it after it arrives. It is far easier to prevent disease than it is to cure or treat it. It is also far less expensive. Some people take better preventive care of their automobile than they do their own body.

In everything that I do I always look for the preventative measures that I can take first. Although there are several other factors, diabetes prevention can be summed up for the most part into four areas: proper diet and weight control, regular exercise, a healthy spine and normal stress levels. If you have these four areas in check, you will drastically reduce your chance of beating or ever getting diabetes.

The Natural Approach

Proper Diet and Weight Control - There are many natural products on the market that help to alleviate the effects of diabetes. There are herbs, homeopathic remedies,

Ayurvedic supplements, and specially formulated drinks that aid in the fight against diabetes.

Let's first look at the help that comes through better eating habits. I think that's the best place to start since most of our problem begins with the fork and spoon. In his book, *The Diabetes Cure: A Natural Plan That Can Slow, Stop, Even Cure Type 2 Diabetes,* Vern Cherewatenko, M.D. writes:

> *For most people with diabetes, weight management can be tricky. As they gain greater control over blood glucose levels, they may find their weight goes up. That's because, in part, they are no longer losing calories in their urine. To maintain their weight, they have to cut the number of calories they were losing before.*
>
> *Here's where using the Food Pyramid and a meal plan comes in. At the very top are fats, oils, and sweets. These should be eaten sparingly by anyone concerned about good health and keeping weight down. Next are dairy and meat/protein. Small amounts of both these areas are necessary, but remember that they're higher in calories than foods at the bottom of the pyramid.[2]*

2. pg 118, c1999 Harper Collins New York, and Paul Perry

In addition to increasing the amount of vegetables and fruits and limiting breads, pastas and cereals, there are also some herbs that you can take that have been useful in helping diabetes. But do your homework and never discontinue diabetic medication without doctor supervison.

...never discontinue diabetic medication without doctor supervison.

When it comes to diabetes, you really can't compromise on diet especially with sugar. Sugar in any form will only increase your glucose levels in an unhealthy and potentially dangerous way. So that means you have to limit bread, pasta and rice, and steer away from bananas, raisins, cakes, pies, cookies, candy, potatoes, and fruit juices like orange juice which contains large amounts of natural sugar. So, you've got the point—NO SUGAR. If you must indulge eat very small portions as they all raise blood sugar significantly. Other things to add to the list of do's and don'ts are. . .

- Decrease all fatty foods (they are high in calories)

- Increase your food intake with low calorie foods (like celery, broccoli and cauliflower)

- More vegetables please. Increase your intake of green vegetables. No fried tomatoes, fried okra, or fried anything for that matter. Frying your vegetables literally takes away the nutrition in them and destroys the enzymes that your body needs. Increase your string beans, onion, and especially garlic consumption. Garlic is a wonder food that helps in stabilizing so many bodily functions and also is instrumental in regulating healthy blood flow to the heart. When you eat salad, be sure to include a healthy portion of cucumbers and a small amount of chicken or fish for added protein.

- As an alternative to sweets, pastries, and sugar-loaded desserts, choose low sugar fruits. Grapefruit is low in sugar and at the same time tastes great. Half an apple makes a tasty snack and helps your gall bladder, too.

- Eat foods in their most natural form to get the full benefit from them. When you eat raw foods they help to stimulate the pancreas and thereby enhance insulin. I know you like the taste and the seasonings, but this is your health that we are talking about, so learn to like new foods. I believe in you, and feel confident that you can do it.

When you feel fatigued, push your way through and begin to do light exercise to increase your metabolism and energy levels. Don't give in to the feeling to lay down or not exercise.

Regular Exercise—I cannot over emphasize the importance and magnitude of getting regular exercise if you are a pre-diabetic, borderline diabetic or been diagnosed as diabetic. Exercise improves circulation, oxygenates tissues, increases flexibility, helps build immunity and strengthens your heart. Most importantly for the diabetic patient, exercise helps to burn off unwanted calories and maintain healthy blood sugar levels.

Importance of a Healthy Spine—We cannot ever dismiss the need for a healthy, strong and well-aligned spine. Your spine is the switchboard to your entire nerve system. Proper alignment of the spine is imperative so that nerve messages can flow freely and uninterrupted to the body and to your pancreas, as well as all of your organs. If a spinal bone becomes subluxated (misaligned) from a sports impact, a slip or fall or a lifting strain, it impedes normal nerve function in whatever organ or body part that the spinal bone is connected to. It works much the same as turning down a dimmer switch dims your dining room light. A properly aligned spine is a precursor to amazing health and well-being in the same way a subluxated, poorly aligned spine is a precursor to poor health and lowered quality of life.

Chiropractors always recommend three things. First, that you get your spine checked (examined), especially if you never have or haven't in the last year or two. This typically involves a consultation, a spinal examination, likely a spinal x-ray and a thermal scan of the spine to check for nerve irritation, postural distortions, muscle contractures and other abnormalities. Second, we recommend that you get all your subluxations corrected, and third, that you keep it that way through regular Chiropractic visits your whole life through.

Someone once said that if your spine were on your face that you would take better care of it.

Think about Chiropractic care like orthodontics for the spine. Someone once said that if your spine were on your face that you would take better care of it. People who do are by far the healthiest people on the planet and incidentally rarely suffer from diabetes.

Your spine is your body's lifeline. People who see their Chiropractor regularly have stronger immune systems, stand straighter, have better balance, perform better athletically, visit doctors less often, take far fewer medications, spend significantly less money on health care and use their insurance much less often.

For a list of some of America's Best Chiropractors personally consult the appendix of this book or for an expanded list, consult the Referral Directory on our website at www.SettingThingsStraight.com.

Relaxation for Stress Reduction—If there is one thing that I really believe everybody needs to do, not only diabetics, is to simply relax. Everybody approaches this area differently. You may choose yoga, watching a movie or television, playing golf, bicycling, swimming, taking a walk, playing tennis, reading a novel or just taking in the sounds of the crashing ocean waves. Whatever it is that you do, do it more often. Relaxation drastically reduces your stress levels hence causing the body to be better able to heal itself. When you are relaxed you can properly assimilate the food, vitamins, minerals, and other supplements that you consume more easily into your bloodstream.

Make the decision now to stop doing all of the things that promote stress in your life. Stay away from stressing people.

Motivation To Start Now

There are many motivations for you to become more aware of your health now and in the last chapter I will discuss how to develop your own unique personal wellness plan. Your main motivation to make conscious choices to improve your health should be that you want to live a fruitful and healthy life. Diabetes is not just a disease that stands alone. It is often the consequence of not taking good enough care of yourself or making your health a top priority. Diabetes is also often a precursor to many other problems in your body. It can cause kidney failure, promote heart disease, slow healing, encourage infections and cause major complications in pregnant women. The good news is that all of those things can be avoided with a little conscious effort. The choice is yours. If you choose not to change you may lose far more than you originally anticipated. Here is what I mean.

Sexual Dysfunction—There are millions of men that wish they made better choices early on that can no longer enjoy sexual intimacy with their partner. It's not widely publicized, but diabetes causes erectile dysfunction in men. Men; is that enough motivation to start? When men get diabetes, a high percentage are affected sexually, as high as 50%.

About half of men with diabetes become impotent. Impotence means that the penis does not become or stay hard enough for sex. There can be a number of causes of impotence another one of which is blood pressure and cholesterol medications. The most common causes of impotence in men with diabetes are:

- *Damage to the nerves in your penis*

- *Damage to the blood vessels in your penis*

- *Poor control over your blood glucose levels[3]*

_____

3. Source: *Diabetes: A to Z What You Need to Know About Diabetes—Simply Put,* Fifth Edition, American Diabetes Association Alexandria, Virginia pg. 159)

Women you are not off the hook. Diabetes also affects female sexuality as well. Women with diabetes often have a loss of sensation, which leads to a total loss of motivation to have sex altogether.

Amputation—There are many other tragic implications of this disease, but one that causes me great concern is the high amount of people that have to get their legs amputated because of this disease. Chronically high blood sugar levels and insulin use can affect circulation and slows healing. This predisposes the limbs especially the legs to swelling, a condition called cellulitis and later to infection which leads to gangrene. Gangrene is death of tissue due to a lack of oxygen and nutrients. Proper and regular foot care is extremely important. Small infections tend to grow rapidly when left unchecked in those prone to sugar regulation problems. Here are some statistics:

Prevention of Amputations

- *67,000 lower limbs are lost yearly in the United States to diabetes-related problems; greater than half of those losses could be prevented with early detection and treatment.*

- *The amputation rate for blacks is 1.5 to 2.5 times greater than whites.*

- *The amputation rater for Native Americans is 3 to 4 times higher than the general population.*[4]

Hopefully you have a better understanding now, about diabetes than you did before you started reading this chapter. As with every chapter in this book, I can only offer you hope for a brighter future. There is no such thing as an incurable disease. However, you do have a role to play in your own healing process. It is true that the physical loss is great particularly when one has loss of a leg, foot or toes. However, the loss is far greater to your family when they cannot enjoy you in your most vibrant and joyous state. Change your mind and choose life!

---

4. Source: pg 233 Cherewatenko

CHAPTER EIGHT

Vitamin Supplements— Where Do I Begin

>—•—<

T he purpose of this chapter is to help to demystify the whole process of choosing vitamins making the procedure far less complicated. One thing that most health practitioners can all agree on is the fact that people need vitamins and supplementation. However, discerning exactly which vitamins we need everyday, from those which we need occasionally, from the ones that we need every once and a while can be pretty wearisome to figure out. If you are anything like me, you love a challenge in life and appreciate a competitive game, but would much rather compete in any area other than the vitamin game. I realize that you can become totally overwhelmed trying to do the right thing, so my aim is to keep it simple.

All kinds of things can go through one's mind when considering vitamins. For example, you may know someone or have a relative that has never taken vitamin supplements in their life and is very healthy. That person could be your grandfather or grandmother, be in their nineties and still going strong. If that is your experience, you might think that the vitamin quest is a worthless pursuit. That's how it may appear to you, but it's just not so. There are always averages, and those that beat the averages in life.

Occasionally someone will beat the odds and live long and healthy without putting any energy or effort into it. They are not the rule but the exception. Most people are not that fortunate. Since the odds are against us we have to make responsible choices to excel in and maintain our health.

You can live without taking vitamins, but I'll guarantee you that you will eventually develop deficiencies in your overall health. Does the brand name count or are all vitamins the same? Is there any quality better than the other? Everybody seems to be pushing their brand, where should I start? I'll answer all of those questions for you just keep reading!

I Hate Pills! Are There Other options?

There was a time when the only option that a person had when it came to taking vitamins was the traditional pill-like format. I realize that many people are just not pill friendly or should I say that many pills are not people friendly. Whatever the case may be, if you don't like pills then you simply are not going to take them.

The good news is that you don't have to. Nobody's forcing you to take those dreadful pills anymore. There are many different options on the market today so that pretty much everybody can take their vitamins one way or another. What matters the most is that you get the supplements in your system. I've listed a few options for you below.

- **Capsules**
- **Chewables**
- **Liquid Vitamins and Minerals**
- **Powdered Vitamins**
- **Tablets**

Synthetic Vitamins VS Natural

Many vitamins are manufactured in a laboratory synthetically and put into pill form and called a vitamin supplement. However, these chemically created vitamins are fake or artificial. The truth is that Vitamin C is

Vitamin C whether it is manufactured in a chemical plant or naturally extracted from a living plant, fruit or vegetable. The difference is that when extracted from a plant, fruit or vegetable it is combined with intrinsic factors. That means that it is not just a raw chemical but is in a sense a live complex of easily absorbed nutrition which your body can readily use.

In the same way that baby formulas are a poor excuse for real mother's milk, synthetic vitamins are poor replicas of Mother Nature's version. It is virtually impossible to tell by looking at a label whether vitamins are real or imposters since the FDA does not require manufacturers to tell you. This is but one more way that the FDA is not doing its part to help support your health and well being.

As a general rule most vitamins that are cheaply priced are synthetic or are made from inferior ingredients. Another rule is that drug stores and large discount chain stores' vitamins are made by drug companies or mass manufacturers. Typically pre-natal and other vitamins that medical doctors prescribe are synthetic and made by drug companies. Typically "one per day" type vitamins also fall into this category. Synthetics are not as easily digested, absorbed, or as usable by the body. So whenever possible buy natural, organic, whole food vitamin supplements.

In most cases the local mom and pop health food store is your best source for whole food, natural vitamins and minerals. Nearly all natural health care providers recommend natural supplements. They do cost a little more but are definitely worth the extra expense.

In addition most natural care providers are well-versed in giving nutritional advice. By consulting them you can make sense out of what to take for your particular and individual needs. This helps to minimize the expense of taking unnecessary supplements and minimizes the total number of daily pills you need to take. For example, a common mistake many of my patients make is to take too many individual supplements when they could take one or two formulas that include everything they need. What too often happens is that friends suggest a specific vitamin for a particular problem such as vitamin E for a skin condition, vitamin A for weak eyes and B6 for Carpal Tunnel Syndrome. All are commonly found in natural combination formulas at your local health food store and therefore costs you less money and makes them easier to take. Let's keep it simple.

Super Foods

In the health food craze of our modern day, you may have heard the phrase super foods or green foods mentioned. There are many different health food brands that sport their own kind of super foods mixture. For the most part super foods are natural whole foods that are easy for the body to digest and assimilate. They also contain a very large amount of nutrients that the body needs. Typically, superfoods are a quick and easy way to get an enormous amount of needed vitamins, minerals, and antioxidants into your blood system.

Some of these super foods are made from alfalfa, algae, barley, wheat grass, pollen and royal jelly. Many manufacturers will blend these foods and other green leafy foods together in a dry mix and package them in containers. I suggest you buy organic super foods which mean they are farmed without artificial chemicals and pesticides.

They suggest that you add fruit juice to one or two scoops daily. It is extremely difficult for you to eat as many vegetables as you need in a day. Super food mixtures have now made it possible for you to get an adequate supply of all of the vitamins, minerals and antioxidants that you need in one easy form. Super foods can be easily mixed into a fruit shake or combined with juicing.

If you don't like shakes, then you may want to use the pill form of super foods. Because the pill is much smaller, you will be required to take a number of pills. Taking your vitamins with some food in your stomach will help you avoid becoming nauseated.

Does Brand Matter?

Let me get right to the point, brands do matter. The old adage, "You get what you pay for," is still a very valid truth. Some people purchase the cheapest quality vitamins that they can find. If you choose that road just to save your money, its better not to buy any vitamins. Usually inexpensive vitamins are manufactured with the lowest quality ingredients, high amounts of additives, sugars, or worse yet, artificial sweetners.

Many of those brands also use synthetic vitamins leaving you with nothing of any real value. At times you may find noted brand names at close out sales and dollar stores. You still need to be careful, as these vitamins may have been shelved for years before they got rescued from the shelves at their former store. Read the label to check if the expiration dates have expired. Freshness is important in supplements, too.

Vitamins that have gone past the expiration date have usually lost their maximum effectiveness. Just because I told you to avoid the cheap stuff does not mean that you have to go broke trying to afford the most expensive vitamins on the market. Don't be fooled on that end either. Just because it's more expensive does not necessarily mean that they are more effective. It may only suggest that the company has higher overhead.

One way to find out how effective vitamins are is by asking people that use vitamins. Word of mouth never fails. If a person is receiving great results from using a particular supplement or company, then it is possible that you may get great results too. Remember though that everybody's body is different. What works for you may not necessarily work for the next person. Understanding your health should be a lifetime journey that you enjoy. You should educate yourself as much as possible. Read printed material about the products that others are asking you to take. Another way to determine if a supplement is good is to let it sit in lukewarm water in a clear glass. Supplements that don't begin to dissolve within 20 minutes or so, may not break down in your body either. Cheap supplements are often pressed into hard capsules and *go* straight through your system and end up in the sewer system.

One warning to you is not to pay much attention to overly advertised products. There are some companies that have a very large advertising budget and can afford to bombard the public with constant commercials and major magazine spreads. That does not always mean that they are better. It just means they have more money to spend. It may very well be possible that a small local vitamin supplier has far better products and quality standards than their big competition, but just do not have the dollars to spend on advertising.

I've found that the better companies typically concentrate on spending more of their dollars on creating a quality product. That makes more sense to me. The bottom line is that the absolute best way to find out which brand is best for you is by trying it for yourself. You may have to do a little searching before you find the brands that are right for you.

General Wellness Supplements Versus Specific Conditions

I am a very strong proponent of getting and maintaining optimum health therefore my approach to supplementation is to consistently cover all of your nutritional bases. You can do that most easily by using a natural multivitamin, mineral and antioxidant formula on a daily basis. This covers a multitude of nutri-

Without a healthy and well-aligned spine it is impossible to have outstanding health.

tional sins. This simple approach goes a long way to preventing deficiencies and supporting your body's ability to heal, repair and rejuvenate itself.

We have talked about the importance of the nervous system in the body and that it coordinates and controls all of the healing in the body. Without a healthy and well-aligned spine it is impossible to have outstanding health.

You become what you eat. The nutrients you take in are the building blocks that your body creates new cells from. Like builders use lumber, bricks and mortar to build a house, your body uses what you eat to recreate you on a regular basis.

It is an incredible testimony to the human body's ability to adapt that it can make eyeballs, toenails, and liver cells from soda, potato chips and French fries. So do your best to avoid ingesting empty calories and food which is void of worthy substance. After all you wouldn't ever build your house out of popsicle sticks and paper mache would you?

Our bodies need a continual source of high quality, nutritional building blocks to create an ongoing vibrant sense of well being.

~

Age Or Condition Appropriate Nutrition

Taking nutrition to the next level would include what I call age or condition appropriate nutrition. This means that I recommend nutrition supplements based on a person's stage of life. For example, men are prone to develop cancer of the prostate. Therefore I recommend a natural prostate support supplement for all men over 50. Many women have sluggish thyroid glands that cause them to easily put on weight, lose their hair, become fatigued, get chilled, lose sex drive and develop dry skin. This is an easy syndrome to spot as a health professional. Thyroid support formulas are easy to find at every good health food store.

Another example would be that everyone in American society is prone to heart disease, clogging of the arteries, stroke, circulation, and blood vessel problems. Flax seed oil, rich in omega 3's, helps to promote healthy cholesterol levels, clean blood vessels, promote joint health, fight arthritis pain and reduce inflammation in the body. Therefore it is one of my best nutritional recommendations. Take 1-2 tablespoons of liquid Flax Seed Oil or equivalent in capsules daily.

Condition Based Nutrition

Another level of nutrition supplementation is condition based nutrition. This gets a little trickier without professional help but there are many good resources available to help you. Recommendations are too vast to list here, yet there are many good resources available to help you. Three suggestions are "Prescription for Natural Cures" by James Balch, M.D. and Mark Stengler, N.D., "Prescription for Nutritional Healing" by James Balch, M.D. and Phyllis Balch C.N.C., and "Natural Cures" by Kevin Trudeau.

On Anxiety, Depression, And Morbid Fears

One area I desperately need to address in this chapter is the growing prevalence of anxiety, panic attacks, depression, crying without reason and unfounded fears that I see in patients. Though there can be other causes which may require medical treatment, these symptoms can commonly be caused by a B complex deficiency.

Stress, sugar intake, and soda all rob the body of precious B vitamins. Prolonged stress and poor diet can finally tip chemical balance in the brain and create psychological and emotional disturbances. This is really scary for the afflicted person. High doses of natural B complex vitamins daily can help restore and normalize the problems. Obviously, immediately eliminating stressors, stressful people and sugar from your life are necessary also.

Not All Calcium Is Created Equally

Perhaps the biggest hoax in the vitamin game is calcium supplements. First of all there is very little evidence that proves that taking calcium prevents or helps osteoporosis. However, until it is proven conclusively that it helps or hinders here is a real important truth to know. Most all calcium supplements are made from calcium carbonate (ie, ground up sea shells or limestone). Calcium carbonate is cheap to make but extremely hard to digest. It takes eight digestive steps to break it down in the body before it can be absorbed and utilized. However, calcium lactate takes only one step. So if you are going to use a calcium supplement, get one made from calcium lactate. It is pennies more expensive but worth it.

Allow me to reiterate some important points. Always use natural, whole food organic supplements whenever possible. Buy at a heath food store. If you are unsure about anything ask the owner who is usually very knowledgeable and can help you sort out the differences. I suggest that you don't ask your medical doctor for nutrition advice as most have little or no nutritional training whatsoever. Ask for recommendations from natural health care experts. A knowledgeable natural health expert can do testing and thorough surveying to determine your specific nutritional needs. They also can offer expert advice and monitoring to help you achieve your health goals.

Avoid buying highly advertised, mass produced vitamins from drug stores and large discount marts. Don't buy the common one per day type supplements or cartoon variety chewable vitamins for your children. Health food stores have fun, great tasting chewables that are far better for your little blessings.

All adults can benefit from a formula containing natural vitamins, minerals and antioxidants. Most should take flax seed oil or fish oil daily. Many would benefit by taking special formulas for specific age related challenges such as thyroid, prostate, female hormone, eyes, etc.

Unfortunately, unless you are living off your own land, growing your own fruits and vegetables, raising your own chickens, eggs, and beef you probably are not getting enough nutrition in your diet. Soil depletion, farming techniques, chemical fertilizers, pesticides, stress and sugar consumption all play a role in sapping nutrition out of your life. So nutrition is a necessary inconvenience.

To close out this chapter, I have listed some of the more common vitamins and their benefits:

- Vitamin A and Beta-Carotene—Helps to maintain healthy skin, treat acne problems, promotes good eyesight, and healthy growth in children.

  Natural Sources: Spinach, carrots, parsley and yams. Also found in egg yolks.

- Vitamin B-1—Promotes tissue healing after surgery. May be used to help prevent Bell's palsy, multiple sclerosis, neuritis, and Alzheimer's disease.

  Natural Sources: Legumes, wheat, rice and oatmeal. Do not overcook any of these foods as it will easily deplete its vitamin content. Vitamin B-1 can also be found in seeds and nuts.

- Vitamin B-2—used in the formation of eye tissues. It helps to relieve stress, fatigue and exhaustion. Works in preventing migraine headaches. May help to prevent intestinal cancer.

  Natural Sources: Brewer's yeast, liver and salmon. Also, found in riboflavin, grains and fruits.

- Vitamin B-3—May help lower cholesterol, metabolizes sugar and reduces allergic reactions.

  Natural Sources: Legumes, whole grains, avocados and dried fruit.

- Vitamin B-5—Helps stress and fatigue related to surgery, illness or injury. Helps to prevent some forms of acne. When taken with vitamin C, it helps to strengthen the skin, promotes the healing of cuts, and increases the flexibility of scar tissue.

  Natural Sources: It is found in most whole foods. But it is commonly found in foods like sweet potatoes, cauliflower, avocados and green peas.

- Vitamin B-6—Is perhaps the most important of all of the B vitamins. Helps to produce energy, good for protein metabolism, and produces healthy nerves.

  Natural Sources: Wheat. Also found in liver and other organs.

- Vitamin B-12—Supports growth, appetite, and red blood cell production. Promotes energy.

  Sources: Only found in animal foods such as dairy products, fish, eggs and meat products.

- Biotin—Helps to metabolize fat and works in synthesizing fatty acids in the body. Helps to maintain healthy hair and skin. Helpful for people with diabetes as it supports fat and carbohydrate metabolism.

  Natural Sources: Rice, egg yolks, yeast. It is also made from your intestinal bacteria.

- Vitamin C—Helps to heal wounds. Supports the immune system. May ward viruses and diseases such as cancer. Protects blood vessels. Keeps body tissues strong. Helps to prevent the common cold. It has been known to help people with cholesterol, cataracts, diabetes, asthma, periodontal disease and various forms of allergies.

  Natural Sources: Most citrus fruits such as oranges, lemons, limes and grapefruit. It is also found in bell peppers, rose hips and strawberries.

- Vitamin D—Helps your body to properly assimilate calcium thus promoting strong bones and may prevent osteoporosis and tooth decay. Typically the greatest benefit comes from this vitamin when it is used with calcium and consistent exercise.

  Natural Sources: Milk, egg yolks, butter and fish.

- Vitamin E—It is theorized that this vitamin helps to protect the reproductive organs. Helps to prevent degenerative diseases of the heart, respiratory system, and the neurological system.

  Natural Sources: Nuts, seeds, whole grains, dark green leafy vegetables, and vegetable oils.

- Folic Acid—Supports metabolic functions such as red blood cell formation, when combined with vitamin B-12. Works in metabolizing protein and amino acid. Folic acid deficiency has been linked to neurological defects.

Natural Sources: Spinach, chard, broccoli, kale, corn, and bean sprouts. One of the best sources is nutritional yeast.

- Inositol—Helps to metabolize fat. Helps prevent cardiovascular disease and viral infections. Supports healthy skin and hair. Some believe that it also helps to increase alertness in patients with Alzheimer's disease.

  Natural Sources: Nuts, wheat germ, molasses, and whole grains.

- Vitamin K—Helps the blood to healthily clot. Supports bone development and helps to prevent osteoporosis.

  Natural Sources: Yogurt, fish oil, eggs and green leafy vegetables.

I recommend taking a natural B complex vitamin formula that includes all of the B vitamins rather than taking an individual B vitamin by itself.

CHAPTER NINE

Conquering Stress the Chiropractic Way

⸻◆⸻

This chapter is dedicated to one of the most horrible inciters of bad health in our modern culture—stress. Everybody has stress. No one is exempt. Stress left unchecked and not dealt with can cause major health complications down the road. What exactly is stress? Stress is literally defined as a force that strains or deforms. Stress can also be defined as a force which puts unnecessary and unhealthy strain on our bodies ultimately negatively affecting our health.

Let's face it, we live in a do more and be more culture. For the most part that is the kind of mentality that traps many of us today. You just purchased a new car last year, but next year's model is completely different than yours. You just moved into the house but a $30,000.00 swimming pool would sure feel nice right about now. The process that we go through in order to get more and be more ultimately puts greater stress on us. Now I'm not suggesting at all, that you should never want to have anything of substance or value in life.

I am trying to convey to you that there are certain things that if understood and avoided would drastically reduce your stress altogether and improve your health. I agree that you need a car, but do you really have to have one every year, especially if that means that you have to compromise your health in order to get it? I would think not.

Great health is equal to real wealth, and you do not have to compromise your health in order to achieve wealth. The get more be more culture is not only stressing our bodies, but our checkbooks as well. So since stress is really something that we need to avoid, let's learn more about how we can effectively deal with this age-old problem.

Different Types Of Stress And Their Causes

There are several kinds of stress. For the most part they all fall under physical, mental-emotional and chemical stresses that people suffer from daily. Physical stress is probably the most obvious stress. You can get physically stressed from lifting something that is too heavy for you to lift, straining yourself. You can get physical stress from an injury, such as a car accident or from repetitive work on an assembly line which causes Carpal Tunnel Syndrome. I care for patients all day long whose bodies are stressed from slumping over a computer for hours on end at their job. These stresses are physical because they are most easily detected in the physical realm.

There is also emotional and mental stress that can be the most deadly of the bunch particularly since its effects cannot always be seen or felt. It is this type of stress that conceals itself for years, maybe even decades seemingly waiting to attack the body in the most violent and catastrophic way. Long-term mental and emotional stress too often manifests itself as cancer, major heart attacks or disabling strokes.

Occupational stress is a combination of physical and mental-emotional stress. For example, police work, nursing, and truck driving are just a few examples of jobs where people have very large responsibilities that carry great pressure. You don't have to be in a life saving or pressure occupation to have occupational stress in your life. Quite obviously police protect the safety of the citizens within a community, through fighting crime. Criminals are diametrically opposed to police and will kill a police officer in a heart beat.

Knowing that you could be killed or injured just for doing your job can definitely bring about great stress.

Nurses and doctors both have the challenge of saving lives. It is always stressful when someone else's life is in your hands. Even Chiropractors deal with the pressure of knowing that our work greatly impacts the outcome of a person's life. Truck drivers live their lives in a constant rush and always have deadlines to meet. When they miss deadlines they are penalized with monetary fines or worse yet, could lose their job.

Although it seems like it should be obvious, there is one kind of stress that many people in society rarely consider and that is chemical stress. While there are ways to protect yourself from getting hurt emotionally, having someone play with your mind, or even, choosing a low-stress job, few people can avoid the overwhelming and invasive presence of chemical stress.

Chemical stress occurs when chemicals in the form of prescription drugs, cigarette smoke, alcohol, and other airborne or food based pollutants and toxins get into your system and alter its ability to perform optimally. This kind of stress is by far the most pervasive killer of them all. It is not always easily detected and can go unnoticed for a very long time. Think about the concept that a person that has never smoked a cigarette can still die from lung cancer, having acquired the disease through second hand smoke. My mother died this way. Let's talk about a major chemical stressor that few people have knowledge of and is one of the world's leading killers.

Drugs Kill

Make no mistake about it, drugs kill people every single day. When I say drugs, I am not limiting drugs to the illegal dealer on the city street corner selling heroin or crack cocaine. I am also referring to the legalized drugs that we can freely buy everyday, the kind that our government gets tax revenues from. Maybe it's just me, but I don't really see a major distinction between the way that the illegal cocaine

Make no mistake about it, drugs kill people every single day.

dealer distributes his or her drugs and the way that the medical and drug industry do it. The only obvious difference is who gets the money and whether you go to jail or not.

I know that some drugs save lives and help people but even marijuana has been hypothesized to cure cancer if you smoke enough of it. The truth as I see it is that if you take responsibility for your own health and make good decisions you will not need legal nor illegal drugs. In my own personal quest for wellness of 34 years I have only received medical care for sickness twice. I needed a prescription medicine one time, for a ten-day period. In all of those years, I have never been hospitalized or diagnosed with a disease. You can be that healthy too.

Drive down any "Main" street in America and you will see all of the drive-through fast-food joints, drive-through beverage distributors, and of course drive-through drug windows. Just think about that for a moment.

The government spends hundreds of millions of dollars policing our borders each year, trying to catch drug dealers and locking them up for their crime. Yet illegal drugs still make it to our streets. Those illegal drugs are responsible for seven thousand deaths annually.

The outrage of modern history is occurring right under our noses.

Worse yet is that the legalized drug business kills far more than the illegal drug business each year. More than one hundred thousand humans die annually from adverse reactions to extreme chemical stress caused by prescribed medication. Some figures suggest that as many as half a million people die annually. Gary Null's study in July of 2004 cited that just less than one million people die yearly from a combination of drugs reactions, medical mistakes, and unnecessary surgeries.

That is a substantial amount of people dying. That number is far higher than it should ever be and it has to stop! The outrage of modern history is occurring right under our noses. More people have died from adverse reaction to drugs than all of the people in the Jewish Holocaust, the African-American slave trade, and the Vietnam War put together. Don't mistake my intentions here. I am not totally against medication. I am grateful for dedicated men and women who work and give their service in the medical field. What I am against is prescription drug abuse, the mongering, and the needless suffering and dying that the government, the medical profession and the drug industry refuse to do anything about. It's all about the money.

If three Airbus Jets were to crash in any 90 day period the FAA and TSA would ground every Airbus Jet until they found and fixed the problem. Yet if Gary Null is right and I believe he is, nearly one hundred thousand Americans will die before the next full moon and nothing is being done about it.

The Silent Killer

As obvious as drug deaths are there is a condition caused by stress that flies under the radar and often goes completely unnoticed. That condition is called a vertebral subluxation. Vertebral subluxation is a medical term which literally means "a minor dislocation of a spinal bone." It is the most common root of illness and by far the most underrated and least investigated health condition that exists.

Vertebral Subluxation was discovered in 1895 by D.D. Palmer in Davenport, IA when he examined the spine of a deaf custodian named Harvey Lillard. Harvey explained that his deafness started 17 years earlier when he was lifting something and felt a pop in his upper spine. When D.D. Palmer examined the area where the pop had occurred he discovered a lump which he surmised was a spinal bone that had become misaligned.

Chiropractic is the fastest growing natural health care profession in the world.

He crudely manipulated the vertebra (spinal bone) back into proper position three times over a period of several days and Harvey's hearing was totally restored. D.D. Palmer's theory, later scientifically proven, was that nerves were being affected at the spine by the misaligned bone. He termed his discovery "Chiropractic" meaning health care "done by hand."

What Is Chiropractic?

Chiropractic is the fastest growing natural health care profession in the world. D.C.'s (Doctors of Chiropractic) specialize in locating and correcting this serious condition known as Vertebral Subluxation. Subluxations occur when an individual does not have their spine regularly checked from birth. They are most commonly caused by stresses and impacts to the body from poor posture, poor sleeping habits, slips and falls, vehicular accidents, sports impacts, strenuous exercise, work injuries, childhood falls, and the birth process. Subluxations cause danger- ous stress to the spinal cord and the delicate spinal nerves as they exit the spine between the spinal bones. This causes irritation to the nerves and affects the body's ability to heal. Nerve interference causes increased sus- ceptibility to disease and disor- der in the body. Unfortunately subluxations are most often painless and often go undetect- ed for years.

It may be obvious that you need to see a Chiropractor if you are experiencing neck pain, back pain, hip pain, headaches, numbness or cur- vature of the spine. However,

Chiropractic treatments called spinal adjustments are safe, gentle, and highly effective.

∼

many people don't realize that chiropractic care has an excellent record of success correcting many health dis- orders as well as helping healthy individuals maintain optimal health. Maintaining a healthy and well-aligned spine is extremely important and is the most overlooked key to staying healthy.

Chiropractic treatments called spinal adjustments are safe, gentle, and highly effective. People of all ages can receive chiropractic care to stay healthy, including infants and the elderly. Years of training, education, and experi- ence enable a Chiropractor to determine how chiropractic care can benefit you and your family. Chiropractors are highly educated, caring professionals sensitive to the natural health care needs of your family.

...the spine is referred to as the lifeline of the human body.

∼

The spine is subject to all forms of stress. Physical stress from birth trauma, body impacts, car accidents, sports injuries, lifting strains and all types of falls can cause the spine to become out of alignment. The muscle strain and tension caused by emotional and mental stress pull abnormally on the supporting tissues of the spine causing vertebral subluxations to occur. Chemical stress from medications, alcohol, cigarette smoke, toxins and pollutants cause subluxations and put stress and strain on our nervous systems. Even eating too much sugar, drinking soda and consuming Trans fats can cause chemical stress and subluxations to the spine.

The reason that chiropractors put so much emphasis on having a strong, healthy, well-aligned spine is because it is the switchboard of the body. The spine is made up of twenty four individual spinal bones. When stacked on top of one another they form a tunnel inside, which the spinal cord runs through. Between each spinal bone is a small hole—one on each side—that nerves exit between. Those nerves, exiting between the 24 spinal bones, extend into a network of more than twelve miles worth of nerves when placed end to end. Someone once said you had a lot of nerve and they were right! Those nerves carry the vital life-giving nerve impulses, which bring your body to life.

Consider someone who has severed their spinal cord in a car accident or diving injury. What happens to their body from that point down? That's right it becomes lifeless. That is the reason that the spine is referred to as the lifeline of the human body. A million or more nerve messages travel down the spine and out over the nerve network everyday at 270 miles per hour. That's faster than Jeff Gordon drives!

If we were to find the spinal nerve that controls the heart and snip it through with a pair of scissors what would happen? You guessed right. The heart would stop because its nerve supply was cut off from the brain. The same is true for any organ in your body.

When a vertebra gets twisted out of its normal proper position it narrows the opening which the spinal nerve passes through. Much like bending a garden hose in half blocks the water coming out of the other end of the hose, subluxations squeeze the nerve. In time the body part or organ that the nerve supplies, stops working properly. It is that simple.

Physical, mental-emotional, and chemical stress cause the spine to subluxate. That subluxation interferes with the brain to body connection and weakness begins. If the condition is left undetected, weakness, then malfunction, sickness, disease and even early death can occur. Subluxations are serious.

Chiropractors Fix Subluxations

The Chiropractor's job is to examine the spine using posture, electronic and thermal imaging and x-ray to detect subluxations in your spine and then to correct them. As a person's spine is re-aligned over time the nerve power is restored to the body and healing can occur. Subluxations block healing. A painless procedure known as a

Research shows that 80% of two year olds have at least one subluxation in their spine.

chiropractic adjustment restores the alignment, releases the irritated nerve and the natural healing ability of the body is restored. Adjustments are most commonly performed by the chiropractor gently pushing on your spine using his or her hands or an adjusting instrument. Sometimes a small, painless popping sensation is felt.

Nearly everyone has subluxations. Research shows that 80% of two year olds have at least one subluxation in their spine. This is most often caused by the modern hospital birthing technique of using the head as handle to twist and pull on the baby's delicate neck. This trauma to a baby's fragile neck and brainstem predisposes many humans to a lifetime of poor health. Many subluxations are also caused by the nearly 1500 falls, which occur during the course of a person's normal experience of learning to walk.

The Solution

It would make very little sense to harp over the many problems in our society and the stressful environment that all of us are subjected to without offering some hope. Getting your spine checked and regularly adjusted by a qualified Chiropractor is the way to vibrant health, decreased sickness and managing stress. I have heard thousands of testimonies over and again abut how people improve their energy, increase their immunity and reduce sickness in their family. Chiropractic has helped people reduce their stress levels drastically. You may ask, "If Chiropractic is all that great then why isn't it more widely accepted?" I'm glad you asked.

The business of treating sickness and disease is big business. It pays to convince people to stay sick even invent new diseases to make people think they are sick. Restless Leg Syndrome, Overactive Bladder and Toenail Fungal Disease are a few new examples. Only sick people take drugs and need medical care. Since Chiropractors represent the very core of health and wellness without drugs or surgery, the Chiropractic profession is fought from literally every angle.

The medical profession has continually fought Chiropractors starting by having Chiropractors thrown in jail in the 1930's for practicing medicine without a license. In the 1960's the AMA (American Medical Association) formed the now infamous committee whose sole intention was to "contain and eliminate the chiropractic profession." In 1981 the AMA was found guilty of violations of the Sherman Antitrust Act against the profession of Chiropractic.

Certain members of the medical profession are still active in underhanded, behind the scenes efforts to undermine the respect for and credibility of Chiropractors. Most recently in Canada and the United States medical exploiters posing as a public interest group are attempting to taint Chiropractic's enormous recent popularity by claiming that Chiropractors cause strokes. There is no evidence to back such claims but that doesn't matter. Their unsubstantiated claims still cause people to fear and live in ignorance. Their efforts are designed to create fear and mis-trust for chiropractic care.

People who live in glass houses shouldn't throw stones. Just today, MSNBC.com news reported that "1.5 million Americans are injured every year by drug errors in hospitals, nursing homes and doctor's offices, a count that doesn't even estimate patient's own medication mix-ups." The article continues on to say, "perhaps the most stunning finding of the report was that, on average a hospitalized patient is subject to at least one medication error per day."[1]

Perhaps the most convincing and hard to dispute argument of the safety of Chiropractic care is the cost of malpractice insurance. Medical doctors pay $40-50,000 per year for malpractice insurance coverage. Surgeons can pay $250,000 or more annually. Chiropractor's malpractice cost is less than $2,000 per year.

The reason is simple. Chiropractors don't kill people. Insurance companies know that we are a safe risk. The medical profession and the drug industry wish we would just go away and the reasoning is pretty clear. As long as we are here and as long as we keep growing in numbers we will eventually saturate the earth with our message of natural wellness without their philosophy and their drugs.

Many people ignorantly believe that chiropractors are only for people who have back or neck pain. Chiropractors are far more than that. In fact, they serve far greater in the area of prevention and wellness. In plain words, by regularly going to your chiropractor and getting adjusted you can totally prevent many health problems and therefore live far healthier than people that do not. Research is scientifically proving what Chiropractors have been preaching since 1895.

---

1. Source: http://www.msnbc.com AP Press July 20, 2006

CHAPTER TEN

Developing Your Personal Wellness Plan—$1 Million Dollar Health Habits

———⋙⋅◆⋅⋘———

First, I really want to congratulate you on your willingness and tenacity to stick it through and read all the way up to this point. I am convinced that you truly want to be healthy. If great health were not your concern you would not have invested so much of you time reading this book. With that in mind, I wanted to let you know that you are well on your way to better health. Although this is the final chapter, it's not the finale. The finale comes when you've implemented one or more of the principles in this work and because of that have experienced healthiness on a totally new level.

Million Dollar Race Horse

I want to ask you a very serious question. If you owned a million dollar racehorse, what would you feed it? Now I am not talking about just any horse here, I am talking about the crème de la crème, the cream of the crop, the best of the best horses ever. You know, the kind of horse that yields you at least one million dollars per race. This horse is a real moneymaker for you. What would you feed your horse? Would you feed it just anything? Would you treat the horse like a nasty old pig and give the horse all of the scraps and leftovers that no one else wanted to eat?

Or would you feed the horse, the best food, the best and most cultured organically grown hay or oats that money could buy? I am sure that you would agree that your horse should eat the absolute best food that you could find. How about exercise? Do you think that you would want to take the horse out every now and again, so that the horse could get some exercise, sunshine, and fresh air? Perhaps you might want to take him out once in a while. Right? Okay, I know that you probably think that I am a bit crazy by now. You are probably thinking, "I'd take my horse out every single day."

And that's absolutely right. You would not only feed your horse the best but you would also make sure that your horse also received an adequate amount of exercise, drank plenty of water, breathed in fresh air and got plenty of sunshine. The reason you would make sure that your horse had the best of everything is because he isn't just any horse. He's not a pony, not a riding horse for little children, and not a horse that simply pulls a buggy around a field. He's a million dollar racehorse. That makes all the difference in the world.

What do million dollars race horses do? They win races. Newsflash! You are the million-dollar racehorse! In fact, you are worth far more than a million dollars, more than billions. So you would not want to treat your own body any less than you would a horse, even if that horse happened to be a million dollar racehorse. I've discovered that most people spend more time and preparation planning their vacation to Disney World, Cancun, or Hershey Park than they do to stay healthy and well. That lack of attention and care for YOU ends right now. You are the most valuable possession in the world. And this personal wellness plan is designed with one intention in mind—WINNING!

Your Personal Wellness Plan

Everybody will have a different wellness plan. Each plan is uniquely tailored to fit the needs of a particular person. What works for me may not work for you and vice versa. But the major point here is that your wellness plan will include you doing something differently than you have before. You will be making one or more changes, trying something new. It may be adding walking to your daily regimen. Perhaps you need to start taking vitamins. Maybe in times past you dreaded drinking water, and now you are up to one eight ounce glass a day.

Whatever the case might be, your wellness plan will definitely include you trying something new for a CHANGE. I have provided a listing of my own personal wellness plan. This may work for you. Or perhaps you may need to tweak it a bit to fit your personal lifestyle. Not only have I provided a list of my plan, but also a list of several sample wellness plans. I'm sure that as you read, you'll begin to catch the idea more clearly of how to personalize your own plan.

Dr. Madeira's Personal Wellness Plan

- Weekly Visit To My Chiropractor
- Take Daily Nutritional Supplements
- Minimum of 7 ½ hours of sleep each day
- 30 minutes of treadmill exercise (3 times a week)
- 15 minutes of light weight lifting (3 times a week)
- Therapeutic massages twice a month for stress management

- Frequent vacations to spend quality time with my family and away from work
- Avoid refined sugar, soda, and trans-fats
- Maintaining a weight of under 170 pounds
- Weekly worship at my church for spiritual growth and enrichment
- Daily devotions which includes Bible reading, prayer, and meditation

A 37 year old husband and father

- Visit the Chiropractor *(weekly)*
- Nutrition Supplements Daily
- Sleep at least 7 hours each day
- 1 hour on the elliptical trainer (daily)
- 15 minutes of light weight lifting (3 times a week)
- 50 Push ups and 100 Sits Ups (daily)
- Avoid medication and medical doctors
- Spend Friday as family night with wife and children
- Listening to spiritual and motivation teaching tapes daily, prayer, regular church attendance
- No red meat

A 29 year old single mom

- Twice monthly visit to the Chiropractor

- Multi-vitamins and minerals
- 8 hours of sleep each night
- Workout at the gym once to twice a week
- Go to the movies once a week for personal enjoyment
- Going out dancing twice a month for stress management and excercise
- Limit soda to one per day
- No French fries or ice cream
- Take the stairs instead of the elevator at work

A 74 year old grandfather

- Weekly Chiropractor visit to align my spine
- Multi-vitamin and fish oil capsules
- Always in bed by 10:00 P.M. each night
- Watch Joel Osteen every Sunday morning at 10:00 A.M.
- 5 minutes of stretching upon rising
- Walk 2 miles everyday outdoors
- Play golf twice a week for relaxation
- Limit Coffee to 2 cups per day

Take time to write your own plan. The key here is that you want to master what you've started. Don't write down 12 things yet only do 2. That'll only discourage you. Write down the things that you are willing to commit to and stick to them. And add another item only after you have mastered the others. My desire for you is not for you to become an overnight success but rather that you will employ successful habits that will last for a lifetime.

...people of faith tend to have lower rates of sickness and degenerative diseases than those that do not embrace faith at all.

You may notice that on each of the personal wellness plans each of them but one has a section devoted to spiritual things, whether it may be attending church or praying or reading the Bible. My purpose here was not to proselytize you but rather to introduce you to a system that is not only working for me but also multiple millions of people all over the world. Studies have shown that people of faith tend to have lower rates of sickness and degenerative diseases than those that do not embrace faith at all. Studies have also shown that prayer is proven to aid in the healing process, even in people with life threatening diseases.

Your body is composed of three major parts. You are body, soul, and spirit. Without getting too complex, basically that means that you have a physical body, a mind, and an inner man or spirit, that I believe is connected to

God. Your body works best when all three components are working together in total harmony as one powerful unit. For example, if you take nutritional supplements every day and exercise, you may think that your physical body is all set, but not so.

You may have an enormous amount of stressfulness, which affects your soul and spirit. In time, that will have an unhealthy affect on your physical body. So everything has to work together all of the time. That's why I believe that a positive mental attitude, prayer, gratefulness and having a sense of living right all affects how you fare in life. It ultimately affects your overall health, performance, and well-being.

How Much Do You Have In Your Account?

Being wellness-minded is a lifelong journey with great rewards. As you are learning about this topic you will instinctively begin to be different based on the new choices that you make. Normally, people that take their health seriously every day tend to keep the bigger picture of life in view at all times. They view their health much like a bank account. With each positive choice you make a deposit into your health account, which by the way earns high dividends.

Every time you go to your Chiropractor for your wellness adjustment you are making another deposit.

Spending more time relaxing, getting more sleep, each night and going for brisk walks or a jog around the neighborhood continually builds interest in your health reservoir. Then when the day comes that you need to take a withdrawal you have something to draw from. I know of many cases where my patient or an acquaintance developed cancer or a heart blockage and needed to get emergency surgery yet survived and recovered quickly and completely, because they took good care of themselves and had a plan and an attitude to stay healthy.

Typically when people age in our society, they get sick, feeble, and diseased. Though that may be characteristic of our society does not make it normal. Many of my senior patients live spry, energetic productive lives. Just this morning, one of my female patients in her seventies, said that her medical doctor couldn't believe that she was her age. At 72 she plays tennis twice each week, rides a motorcycle, and takes no prescription medication.

When asked, "How do you do it"? She credits her healthy state to regular chiropractic care, careful diet, energetic lifestyle, and having a positive mental attitude. That is her personal wellness plan in a nutshell, and it's obviously working well for her. But more than that her commitment to healthy living and making consistent deposits into her account will assure that she will be fine in the rare event that sickness comes her way. Her deposits will support her. It's no different than a person who has been saving money consistently since they were in the early twenties, and then in their winter years, they have a fortune to feast from. What you do today, will have a drastic affect on your tomorrow.

My seventy-year-old patient's story is not the only one. In the past year I lost my two oldest patients. One was 103 years old when he passed, and the other was 96. Both of them were in excellent health and lived long and fulfilled lives. They really only experienced a health breakdown the last 30 days of their lives—not bad after 100 years. When they died neither of them experienced any pain. Martha, the 96-year-old woman had been receiving regular chiropractic for as long as she could remember. Monte, the 103-year-old man started receiving Chiropractic care at the age of 97. That spoke volumes to me about how much he valued his health.

"A Healthy Spine Means A Healthy You."

She loved seeing her Chiropractor. Both of them realized how well spinal care works to maintain good health. I've always said, "A Healthy Spine Means A Healthy You." How much do you have in your account? If you found out that you had a serious disease would your body have the ability to fight off the disease based on your healthy deposits over the years, or would you die in the fight. Again, I say you don't have to do everything in one shot. It's not about how many things you do, but rather how often you do the things you should do. How much money would you have if you took one penny and doubled it every day for a year? You think 365 cents, 365 dollars. Wrong both times.

You'd have more than a million dollars because of the effects of compounded interest. Compounded interest works the same way with your body. Double your ability, double your knowledge about health, double your exercise, or any other area you may need to double, and in time you will have million dollar health.

We All Have To Go Sometime

Many people use the excuse for having bad health habits, "Well we all have to go sometime, so I might as well enjoy myself while I'm here." I fully agree with you. But just because we all will inevitably die doesn't mean that we should live our life recklessly or carelessly and die before our appointed time. You can have an incredibly enjoyable life without being abusive to your body. Just like you can drive a car without abusing it, your body will go a long distance if you make a conscious choice to treat it better.

When you die, and hopefully that's a long time from now, I want you to die healthy, not sick. Unfortunately, most people get sicker and sicker with each sickness or disorder that comes into their system. It's almost as if one thing leads to another and the power of compounded interest begins to work adversely in the body and produces more sickness, then disease and death.

A normal healthy life is one where you are well enough to enjoy living...
～

A normal healthy life is one where you are well enough to enjoy living and you are tapping into your spiritual, social, and emotional potential, living life to the fullest. To leave this world healthy you must have a plan, which consists of a set of quality healthy principles that you live by. That's what a personal wellness plan is all about. The average American dies from one of 3 causes: heart disease, cancer, or an adverse reaction to prescription drugs. In fact, 4 out of every 6 die from one of those causes each year, which is absolutely insane.

In this book, I've given you numerous options to implement into your wellness plan. Anyone that follows the plan that I've mapped out in this book would rarely die from heart disease, cancer or from a stroke. Nor would they ever likely die from a drug reaction, because they wouldn't need to take them. That's good news! The sad news is that you will die from something. But when you do I trust that you will leave this earth when you are really supposed to and not before: to spend eternity with Jesus. Go in God's timing, God's way, not with suffering and pain and live life out loud.

We all have to go, and I've got to leave you now so I can get back and help my patients to live optimal lives. Don't worry; I'll be back with a sequel to this work to help you to continue your pursuit of health, happiness, and the good life. Until next time, work your plan and watch a totally new you arise.

SETTING THINGS STRAIGHT PROVIDERS

These Doctors Represent Some of the
Best Chiropractors in North America

Arizona

Mike Henriksen, D.C.
Spinal Correction Center
1327 E. Chandler Blvd
Suite #106
Phoenix, AZ 85048
(480) 460-1177
www.spinalcorrectioncenter.com
turbo3d1@cox.net

Colorado

Mark L. Botha D.C.
Kristina R. Ring, D.C.
Botha Chiropractic
159 Madison Street
Denver, CO 80206
(303) 321-2252
www.bothachiropractic.com
bothachiro@yahoo.com

Jerry B. Guevara
1231 Lake Plaza Drive
Colorado Springs, CO 80906
(719) 576-2225
jbguevara@adelphia.net

Nate Irwin, D.C.
Irwin Family Chiropractic
2531 S. Shields St., Suite 2J
Fort Collins, CO 80526
(970) 472-8333
www.irwinfamilychiropractic.com
irwinfamilychiropractic@yahoo.com

Ian L. Jones III, D.C.
Creekside Chiropractic
Wellness Center

7596 W. Jewell Ave. Ste. 302
Lakewood, CO 80232
(303) 980-1298
www.drijones.com

Daniel Knowles, D.C.
Richelle Knowles, D.C.
Network Family Wellness Center
1715 15th Street
Boulder, CO 80302
(303) 998-1000
www.networkwellnesscenters.com
frontdesk@networkwellnesscenters.com

Michael Madden, D.C.
Broadway Chiropractic Center
544 S. Broadway
Denver, CO 80209
(303) 733-3522
www.chiropracticcolorado.com

Florida

Mickey Cohen, D.C.
Nob Hill Family Chiropractic
1848 N. Nob Hill Rd
Plantation, FL 33322
(954) 476-8884
www.Nobhillchiropractic.com
NobFamChiro@aol.com

Robert E. Davis III, D.C.
Davis Family Chiropractic
6700 Winkler Road, Suite #3
Fort Myers, FL 33919
(239) 482-8686
www.Chiropractic-Florida.com
drdavis@chiropractic-Florida.com

James Ryan Fenn, D.C.
Fenn Chiropractic Health &
Wellness
2732 Capital Circle N.E.
Tallahassee, FL 32308
(850) 386-7700
www.fennchiro.com
fennchiro@hotmail.com

Christopher W. Hood D.C.
E. Danielle Hood, D.C.
Hood Family Chiropractic Center
5990 54th Ave. N.
St. Petersburg, FL 33709
(727) 544-9000
www.hoodchiropractic.com
info@hoodchiropractic.com

Jeremiah Joseph, D.C.
Kristin Klopfer Joseph, D.C.
Chiro-Med Health and Rehab
655 N. Indiana Avenue, Suite A
Englewood, FL 34223
(941) 473-7900
www.Chiromedhealthandrehab.com
Chiro-medhealthandrehab@veri-
zon.net

Jana Lampe, D.C.
Lampe Family Chiropractic
4144-2 Cleveland Ave.
Ft. Myers, FL 33901
(239) 939-9796
www.drlampe.com
www.info@drlampe.com

Michael Lampe, D.C.
Lampe Family Chiropractic
601 Del Prado Blvd. N#5
Cape Coral, FL 33909
(239) 573-7988
www.drlampe.com
www.info@drlampe.com

Chaz McCants, D.C.
McCants Chiropractic
Wellness Center
4881 NW 8th Ave., Suite 3
Gainesville, FL 32605
(352) 374-0940
drchaz10@yahoo.com

Jeffrey E. Raheb, D.C.
Raheb Family Chiropractic
6705 38th Ave. N., Suite B
St. Petersburg, FL 33710
(727) 381-3456
www.rahebchiropractic.com
Rahebchiro@yahoo.com

Michael J. Risoldi, D.C.
Risoldi Family Chiropractic
25845 US Hwy. 19 N
Clearwater, FL 33763
(727) 797-9900
www.risoldi.com
drmike@risoldi.com

Bret Scheuplein, D.C.
Park Lake Chiropractic
300 E. Colonial Dr.
Orlando, FL 32801
(407) 839-1045
www.ParkLakechiro.com
Bscheup@yahoo.com

Illinois

Luke Lotriet, D.C.
Lotriet Family Chiropractic
13717 South US RT 30
Suite 12
Plainfield, IL 60544
(815) 327-3540
www.drlukel.com
lotrietchiro@hotmail.com

Melvin J. D'Souza, D.C.
804 W. 31st Street
Chicago, IL 60608
(312) 842-2447
melvin@drdsouza.com

Kansas

Matthew Gianforte, D.C.
Meredith Gianforte, D.C.
LifeWorks Chiropractic
22223 W 66th St.
Shawnee, KS 66226
913-397-2293
www.lifeworkschiro.com
drmatt@lifeworkschiro.com

Appendix of Chiropractors

Kentucky

Jacob Bullock, D.C.
  Bullock Family Chiropractic
  2387 Professional Heights Dr.
  Suite 180
  Lexington, KY 40503
  (859) 272-0099
  www.BullockFamilyChiropractic.com
  bullockchiropractic@yahoo.com

Louisiana

Patrick Ford, D.C.
  2325 Severn Ave., Suite 3
  Metairie, LA 70001
  (504) 828-5285
  pforddc@hotmail.com

Phillip L. Smith, D.C.
  Smith Chiropractic Center
  525 E. New River St., Suite B
  Gonzales, LA 70737
  (225) 644-8671
  www.drphilfamilydc.com
  drphil@eatel.net

Maryland

Todd Winebrenner, D.C.
  Winebrenner Spine & Wellness
  4500 Black Rock Road, Suite 103
  Hampstead, MD 21074
  (410) 239-4000
  www.drtoddw.com
  drtodd@drtoddw.com

Massachusetts

William Bazin, D.C.
  Bazin Chiropractic Office
  200 N. Main Street
  Suite 10
  East Longmeadow, MA 01028
  (413) 525-2932
  www.bazinchiro.com
  bazinchiro@aol.com

Mark Potter, D.C.
  366 Massachusetts Ave.
  Suite 103
  Arlington, MA 02474
  (781) 648-8500
  drp@drmarkpotter.com

Kevin Morey, D.C.
  Morey Family Chiropractic
  90 Main Street
  Leominster, MA 01453
  (978) 534-9500
  www.moreyfamilychiro.com
  drmorey@moreyfamilychiro.com

Michigan

Tom Klapp, D.C.
  First Choice Chiropractic
  4748 Washtenaw Ave.
  Ann Arbor, MI 48108
  (734) 434-1100
  www.firstchoicechiropractic.com
  tomklapp@firstchoicechiropractic.com

Jacqueline Vaughn, D.C.
Ronda Vaughn Marshall, D.C.
  Vaughn Chiropractic
  3093 Sashabaw Suite B
  Waterford, MI 48329
  (268) 674-4898
  www.drvaughnmarshall.com
  roniv79@sbcglobal.net

Minnesota

Anthony Lambert, D.C.
  Lambert Family Chiropractic
  1320 South 3rd Street, W
  Missoula, MT 59801
  (406) 541-9355
  www.lambertfc.com
  info@lambertfc.com

Missouri

Jason Harre, D.C.
  Harre Family Chiropractic
  869 St Fancois Street
  Florissant, MO 63031
  (314) 839-8884
  www.drjason.org
  fvcc@charter..net

Nebraska

Charles W. Schollmeyer, D.C.
   1920 North Bell St.
   Fremont, NE 68025
   (402) 721-5500
   doc@schollmeyer.com

New Jersey

Nicola Bonner, D.C.
   Healing Hands of Manahawkin
   588 E Bay Ave Unit 1
   Manahwkin, NJ 08050
   (609) 978-4304
   www.drnicolebonner.com
   HealingHandsofManahawkin@veri-
   zon.net

James Galgano, D.C.
Antoinetta Sorbara D.C.
   Burlington Chiropractic
   321 West Broad Street
   Burlington, NJ 08016
   (609) 747-1100
   www.Burlingtonchiro.com

Jodi Kinney, D.C.
   Intrinsic Chiropractic Center
   100 W. Veterans HWY.
   Jackson, NJ 08527
   (732) 833-9000
   www.intrinsicchiro.com
   drjodi@intrinsicchiro.com

Kimberly Maziarz-Carlucci, D.C.
   Chiropractic Family Health
   86 Valley Rd
   Montclair, NJ 07042
   (973) 744-9880
   drkimmymaz@aol.com

Anita L. Mihlon, D.C.
   Mihlon Family Chiropractic Center
   709 Route 9
   Bayville, NJ 08721
   (732) 237-0933
   www.mihlonchiropractic.com
   dranita@mihlonchiropractic.com

Joseph J Nappi, D.C.
   82 Bethany Rd
   Hazlet, NJ 07730
   (732) 888-1444
   napjacs@optonline.net

Jody L. Serra, D.C.
   Center for Natural Health
   1386 Route 22 West
   Lebanon, NJ 08833
   (908) 236-6353
   www.lesspainbetterhealth.com
   jodyserra@hotmail.com

New Mexico

Craig B. Cathey, D.C.
   Cathy Chiropractic
   713 W. Alameda Street
   Roswell, NM 88203
   (505) 622-0902
   craigcathey@yahoo.com

New York

Randal R. Boivin, D.C.
   Upstate Chiropractic
   138 East Genesee Street
   Baldwinsville, NY 13027
   (315) 635-2333
   www.upstatechiro.com
   randyboivin@yahoo.com

Douglas K. Sullivan, D.C.
   B.C. Family Chiropractic
   3660 George F. Hwy
   Endwell,NY 13760
   (607) 754-5900
   www.bcchiropractic.com

Chad Wells, D.C.
Leah Wells, D.C.
   Wells Family Chiropractic, PLLC
   1116 State Route 434
   Owego, NY 13827
   (607) 687-8787
   www.wellsfamilychiropractic.com
   wellsfamilychiropractic@yahoo.com

Appendix of Chiropractors

North Carolina

Traci Miller, D.C.
Healthy Living Chiropractic
17228 Lancaster Highway,
Suite 208
Charlotte, NC 28277
(704) 271-3160
kidschiro@carolina.rr.com

Bryan G. Ruocco, D.C.
Adjusting the World
16419-C Northcross Drive
Huntersville, NC 28078
(704) 895-7227
adjustingtheworld@yahoo.com

Donald R. Acton, D.C.
Acton Family Chiropractic
789 Patton Avenue
Asheville, NC 28806
(828) 258-0264
www.actonfamilychiros.com

Ohio

Robert DeMaria, D.C.
North Coast Chiropractic
Drugless Health Care
362 E. Bridge Street
Elyria, OH 44035
(440) 322-3418
www.drbob4health.com
druglesscare@aol.com

Pennsylvania

Jack Herd, D.C.
Brian T. Carver, D.C.
Herd Chiropractic Clinic
2704 Market Street
Camp Hill, PA 17011
(717) 737-1681
www.herdclinic.com
herdclinic@aol.com

Christine L. Curran, D.C.
Cornerstone Chiropractic LLC
11 U.S. Route 15 North #6
Dillsburg, PA 17019

(717) 432-4336 or
(717) 421-8842
drchristine.curran@gmail.com

Pamela Dunn, D.C.
33 A East Simpson Street
Mechanicsburg, PA 17055
(717) 697-9100
www.drsdunn.com
drdunn@paonline.com

Zoltan Fischer, D.C.
Fischer Chiropractic
6716 Frankford Avenue
Philadelphia, PA 19135
(215) 333-1915
www.drzoltanfischer.com
drzolfi@verizon.net

Donald P. Henriques, D.C.
Dynamic Chiropractic P.C.
626 Peach Alley South
Elizabethtown, PA 17022
(717) 367-6224
www.drdononline.com
dynamicchiropractic@earthlink.net

Tom Horn, D.C.
Horn Family Chiropractic
8 State Street
Towanda, PA 18848
(570) 265-9796
www.familydc.com
familydc@epix.net

Charisse J. Huston, D.C.
Huston Family Chiropractic &
Wellness Center
6100 Jonestown Rd., Suite A
Harrisburg, PA 17112
(717) 541-9668
www.drhuston.com
doccjh@msn.com

Matthew J. Joseph, D.C.
Walnut Street Wellness Center
40 S. Walnut Street
Sharpsville, PA 16150
(724) 962-5025
josephchiro@yahoo.com

Jeff Ludwick, D.C.
    Camp Hill Family Chiropractic
    3401 Hartzdale Drive, Suite 117
    Camp Hill, PA 17011
    (717) 761-8840
    www.drludwick.com
    jaludwick@hotmail.com

Ross D. Lyon, D.C.
    A.B.E. Chiropractic Center
    1618 Schadt Avenue
    Whitehall, PA 18052
    (610) 433-2656
    www.drrosslyon.com
    drrossdlyon@aol.com

Scott Maclary, D.C.
Christine Maclary, D.C.
    Maclary Family Chiropractic
    402 South Broad Street
    Lititz, PA 17543
    (717) 625-2223
    www.maclarychiro.com
    maclarychiro@dejazzd.com

David Madeira, D.C.
Angela Madeira, D.C.
    Madeira Chiropractic Center
    114 Prince Street
    Harrisburg, PA 17109
    (717) 545-4545
    drdavemadeira@comcast.net

Julie Madeira Niedwick, D.C.
    Madeira Chiropractic
    2507 Gettysburg Road
    Camp Hill, PA 17011
    (717) 766-9700
    www.docjulie.com
    jmadnied@paonline.com

Leo McCormick, D.C.
Darryl Hajduczek, D.C.
    McCormick Chiropractic
    92 Kemp Road
    Pottstown, PA 19465
    (610) 705-0201
    www.mccormickchiropractic.com
    l.mccormick@att.net

Michael D. Morrison, D.C.
    Advance Care Chiropractic
    1205 W. Market Street
    Lewisburg, PA 17837
    (570) 523-1221
    dr_moe7@yahoo.com

Tana M. Nazar, D.C.
    Nazar Chiropractic Family
    Health Center, P.C.
    4800 Derry Street
    Harrisburg, PA 17111
    (717) 564-1550
    www.drtananazar.com
    nazarchiro@aol.com

John Madeira, D.C.
Kelli M. Ross, D.C.
    Madeira Chiropractic
    158 W. Caracas Avenue
    Hershey, PA 17033
    (717) 533-6100
    www.drmad.com
    drmad@comcast.net
    kmrdc@entermail.net

Jeremiah D. Schreiber, D.C.
    River of Life Chiropractic
    2104 Zimmerly Road
    Erie, PA 16509
    (814) 866-2277
    www.riveroflifechiropractic.com
    drjerdc@velocity.net

Darryl Warner, D.C.
    Warner Family Chiropractic
    201 Hospital Drive
    Everett, PA 15537
    (814) 623-5592
    docdkw@aol.com

Dean E. Boyer, D.C.
Matt E. Boyer, D.C.
    217 Point Township Drive
    Northumberland, PA 17857
    (570) 473-3585
    dbcc@chilitech.net

Benjamin M. Grisafi, D.C.
    Grisafi Chiropractic
    507 W. Germantown, Pike
    Norristown, PA 19403

(610) 275-3355
www.drgrisafi.net

Sharon R. Gorman, D.C.
 Gorman Chiropractic Life Center
 9 Crystal Street
 East Stroudsburg, PA 18301
 (570) 476-4100
 www.gormanchiropractic.com

David S. Parker, D.C.
 Family Tree Chiropractic
 904 Dawn Avenue
 Ephrata, PA 17522
 (717) 738-2555
 familytreechiropractic@hotmail.com

Selina Sigafoose-Jackson, D.C.
Kevin Jackson, D.C.
 Sigafoose & Jackson Chiropractic
 2816 E. Market Street
 York, PA 17402
 (717) 757-5731
 www.sigafoosejackson.com
 sig-jack@hotmail.com

South Carolina

Marvin Arnsdorff, D.C.
 Chiropractic USA
 1004 Anna Knapp Blvd, Suite 1
 Mt. Pleasant, SC 29464
 (843) 881-0046
 www.backpacksafe.com
 www.chiropracticusasc.com

Tennessee

Dale Smith, D.C.
Carol Smith, D.C.
 Smith Chiropractic Clinic
 1620 Bonnie Lane, Suite 106
 Cordova, TN 38016
 (901) 794-0876
 www.smithchiropracticcordova.com
 docmom93@aol.com

Texas

Laura Le, D.C.
Steven Le, D.C.
 Stonecreek Family Chiropractic

2200 Morriss Rd., Suite 200
Flower Mound, TX 75028
(972) 874-7554
www.doctorle.com
stonecreekfamilychiropractic@
hotmail.com

John J. Madden, D.C.
 Madden Family Chiropractic
 1201 S. I-35 Suite 103
 Round Rock, TX 78664
 (512) 255-0401
 www.chiropractictexas.com
 jmadden27@yahoo.com

Nikisha T. McDaniel, D.C.
 Magnolia Chiropractic, P.A.
 1430 N. MacArthur Blvd.,
 Suite 104
 Irving, TX 75061
 (972) 554 1511
 www.magnolia-chiropractic.com
 dr.mcdaniel@
 magnolia-chiropractic.com

Terry A. Smedstad, D.C.
 Woodway Wellness Family
 Chiropractic
 4801 Woodway 175 E
 Houston, TX 77056
 (713) 622-2225
 dr.smedstad@yahoo.com

Washington

Jeff A. Sullivan, D.C.
 Diamond Chiropractic
 294 Torbett St.
 Richland, WA 99354
 (509) 943-5533
 www.diamondchiro.com

Canada

Michael Reid, D.C.
Lise Cloutier, D.C.
 209-1419 Carling Ave.
 Ottawa, ON K1Z 7L6
 (613) 761-1600

IF YOU ENJOYED THE BOOK,
YOU WILL LOVE THE:

Setting Things Straight
"30 Minute Wellness Workshops"
By John Madeira, D.C.

30 Minute Wellness Workshops Audio CD Titles Include:

1. "How to Improve Your Energy by 100%"

2. "Losing Weight the Natural Way"

3. "How to Boost Your Immune System"

4. "Preventing Cancer Naturally Before it Begins"

5. "Enhancing Your Body's Healing Power"

6. "Lowering Cholesterol Naturally Without Drugs"

7. "The Chiropractic Answer to Stress"

8. "Developing Your Personal Wellness Plan"

ORDER YOUR COPIES TODAY AT

www.SettingThingsStraight.com

North America's Best Chiropractors

"Set Things Straight" in your life and get on the road to a healthier you! For a list of some of North America's Best Chiropractors please see the appendix of this book. For an updated list and website links please visit:

www.SettingThingsStraight.com

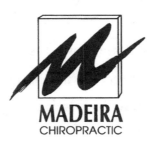

MADEIRA
CHIROPRACTIC

To schedule an appointment at the Madeira Chiropractic Wellness Center in Hershey, PA USA please call (717) 533-6100.

Madeira Chiropractic Wellness Center
158 Caracas Avenue
Hershey, PA 17033
(717) 533-6100 www.DrMad.com

PUBLIC APPEARANCES & CORPORATE EVENTS

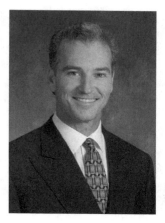

Dr. Madeira is available on a limited basis to speak at your next Corporate Event or Convention. His energetic speaking style will inspire, educate and motivate your employees or downline to greater levels of health, wealth and personal confidence.

To schedule or inquire about a Television, Radio or Corporate Appearance, please contact Joyce Kapp at (877) 623-3472 or visit www.SettingThingsStraight.com

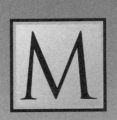